ABOUT THE AUTHOR

As well as being a novelist, Nicci Gerrard is a journalist, a campaigner and a humanist celebrant. In 2016 she won the Orwell Prize for Journalism, for 'Exposing Britain's Social Evils', with a piece exploring the 'language' of dementia.

Following her father's terrible final year and his death in November 2014, she and her friend Julia Jones founded John's Campaign, which insists that the carers of people with dementia have the same right as parents of sick children to accompany them when in hospital. The campaign, which seeks to make care for those who are vulnerable and powerless more compassionate, began in a kitchen but is now a national movement, recognized by NHS policy-makers, by charities, by nurses and by doctors and carers. Four hundred hospitals have already signed up to the campaign.

PENGUIN BOOKS

WHAT DEMENTIA TEACHES US ABOUT LOVE

'An extraordinarily luminous book, at once terribly sad and frightening but also somehow hopeful and energising' Nick Duerden, *i newspaper*

'A profoundly moving elegy ... offers a message of hope' *Daily Mail*

'An incisive and compelling read. Gerrard, a crime novelist and former journalist, visits the "fresh hell" of hospitals across the UK, and interviews sufferers and those whose lives have been indelibly shaped by the diagnosis of a loved one ... Gerrard has personal experience of the creeping attrition that defines this sickness. She watched as the disease slowly and silently insinuated itself into her family's life ... As well as being part-memoir and part-reportage, *What Dementia Teaches Us about Love* is also a great part philosophical inquiry into the nature of self and what it is to be human' Helen Davies, *Sunday Times*

'Gerrard ranges widely and wisely, raising questions about what it is to be human and facing truths too deep for tears' Blake Morrison, poet and author of *And When Did You Last See Your Father?*

'This is a tender, lyrical, profound, urgent book ... Gerrard has penned a treatise on what it is to be human' Yasmin Alibhai-Brown

'Evocative and powerful, shining a light on a world which is often hidden and misunderstood' Jane Cummings, Chief Nursing Officer for England

'A sensitive investigation into dementia based on the author's own experiences as her father was taken by the creeping attrition of the sickness' *Sunday Times* 100 Best Summer Reads

'Gerrard writes beautifully, encyclopaedically and with humanity' Nicholas Timmins, senior fellow at the Institute for Government and the King's Fund, honorary fellow of Royal College of Physicians, author of *Five Giants*

'Nicci Gerrard exudes understanding of the breadth, scale and complexity of the dementias and the challenges they pose for society. Yet she communicates simply, personally and practically as if speaking individually to each of us' Sebastian Crutch, Professor of Neuropsychology, Dementia Research Centre, University College London

'Nicci Gerrard writes with power, insight, empathy and extraordinary beauty about the world of dementia ... and demonstrates how we can address the fear, despair and ignorance that has accompanied its spread' Paul Webster editor of the *Observer*

NICCI GERRARD

What Dementia Teaches Us about Love

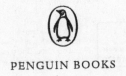

PENGUIN BOOKS

PENGUIN BOOKS

UK | USA | Canada | Ireland | Australia
India | New Zealand | South Africa

Penguin Books is part of the Penguin Random House group of companies
whose addresses can be found at global.penguinrandomhouse.com

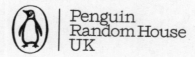

First published by Allen Lane 2019
Published in Penguin Books 2020
001

Typeset by Jouve (UK), Milton Keynes

Printed and bound in Great Britain by Clays Ltd, Elcograf S.p.A.

A CIP catalogue record for this book is available from the British Library

ISBN: 978-0-141-98643-2

www.greenpenguin.co.uk

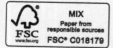

MIX
Paper from
responsible sources
FSC® C018179

Penguin Random House is committed to a
sustainable future for our business, our readers
and our planet. This book is made from Forest
Stewardship Council® certified paper.

To John Gerrard: Letting Go

(And to Patricia Gerrard, Jackie Gerrard-Reis, Tim Gerrard, Katie Jackson: with gratitude and enduring love)

'Abyss has no Biographer'

– Emily Dickinson

Contents

Beginnings

'O the mind, mind has mountains; cliffs of fall
  Frightful, sheer, no-man-fathomed . . .'

The year before my father died, he came with us to Sweden for the summer. He had been living with his dementia for over ten years by then, and – mildly, sweetly, uncomplainingly – he was gradually disappearing, memories falling away, words going, recognition fading, in the great unravelling. But he was very happy on that holiday. He was a man who had a deep love for the natural world and felt at home in it; he knew the names of English birds and insects, wildflowers and trees. When I was a child, I remember him taking me to listen to the dawn chorus in the woods near our house. Standing under the canopy of trees in the bright wash of sound, he would tell me which song was the mistle thrush and which the blackbird. At least, I think I remember this, but perhaps I make it up as a story to tell myself when I'm sad.

In Sweden, he picked wild mushrooms in the forest, went to a joyful crayfish party where he drank aquavit and wore a garland in his white hair, sat with a palette of watercolours looking out at the meadow although his paintbrush never quite made it to the paper. And one evening, we took him to have a sauna – he loved saunas because they reminded him of the time he had spent in Finland as a carefree young man. Afterwards, we helped him into the lake. It was a beautiful, soft dusk; in the fugitive light, the trees were massed shapes and there was a moon shining on the water. I remember the stillness, just the occasional lap of water against the jetty.

My father, old and frail, swam out a few yards and then he started to sing. It was a song I'd never heard before, have never heard since. He was swimming in small circles and singing to himself. He seemed quite contented, happy even, but at the same time it was the loneliest sight: as if there was no one left in the world, just him in the half-darkness and brimming silence, with the lake and the trees and the moon and scattered stars.

The edges of the self are soft; the boundaries of the self are thin and porous. In that moment, I could believe that my father and the world were one; it was pouring into him, and he was emptying out into it. His self – bashed about by the years, picked apart by his dementia – was, in this moment of kindness, beyond language, consciousness and fear, lost and contained in the multiplicity of things and at home in the vast wonder of life.

Or that is what I tell myself now, three years later, trying to make sense of an illness that has the power to dismantle the self, that comes like a robber in the night to sneak into a house built up over a lifetime, to wreck and plunder and despoil it, sniggering behind the broken doors. The following February my father went into hospital with leg ulcers that were slow to heal. There were strict visiting hours and then, with an outbreak of norovirus, a virtual lockdown of the ward, which meant that for days on end he was alone: nobody to hold his hand, speak his name, tell him he was loved; nobody to keep him tethered to the world. His leg ulcers were healed, but away from the home he loved, stripped of familiar routines and surrounded by strangers and machines, he swiftly lost his bearings and his fragile hold upon his self. There is a great chasm between care and 'care', and my father fell into it.

When he at last came home, he was a ghost of himself, skeletal, immobile, inarticulate and lost. No more saunas for him, no more forests and lakes and flowers in his hair; he wasn't in the twilight of the illness now but in its gathering dark. After several months of radically slowed-down dying, as autumn turned to winter and with a hard cold wind blowing, he left us at last. But against the memories of his terrible last months – the small room downstairs where he lay in a hospital bed waiting and waiting for nothing while the birds he loved came to the bird table outside his window; the routine of washing, feeding, lifting; the nurses and doctors and carers and the whole bureaucracy of illness and death; the sense of a mind dying and a body crumbling and not a damn thing to be done about it – against this stifling, drawn-out ending, I set the memory of my father in a Swedish lake, in peace, in soft dusk and that mysterious fusion of the self with the world.

I used to say that we are made of our memories, but what happens when memories are lost? Who are we then? If we are out of our mind, where have we gone? If we have lost the plot, what happens to the story we are in? Even at the bitter end, I never thought my father wasn't himself – although at the same time I felt he had lost himself. He was gone but he remained; he was absent and yet powerfully present. There was something that endured beyond language and recollection, a trace perhaps, like grooves that life had worn into him the way a river carves into rock. He still had his sweetness; his past lived on in his smile, his frown, the way he raised his bushy silver eyebrows. It lived on in us. He might not have recognized us, but we could recognize him. I don't know what the word for this indelible essence is – once, it would have been 'soul'.

Civilization, control and safety form a crust over deep waters. In all of us, often pushed into the corner of our minds, is the uneasy awareness of how frail our hold over ourselves is, how precarious a grip we have on our own minds and bodies. Dementia – all the many and often harrowing forms of dementia – makes us ask what is it to be a self, to be human.

It is often called the plague of our time; it is the 'disease of the century'.

In 2015, an estimated 850,000 people in the UK were living with a form of dementia; the same number was thought to be undiagnosed. As the population ages, it is estimated this figure will increase to over 1 million by 2021 and 2 million by 2051. In the US, the estimate in 2017 was 5.5 million people. According to the World Health Organization, there are around 47 million people living with dementia in the world. Someone develops dementia every three seconds.

People talk of dementia as if it were a time bomb. In truth, the bomb went off long ago, but quietly, privately, out of sight: a hidden demolition job. Men and women who live with dementia are often missing people – forgotten and denied by a society that values independence, prosperity, youth and success and turns away from vulnerability. They are the reminders that we get old, we decay; death comes to us all in the end. Of all the illnesses, it is the one we now most fear. It is 'the story of suffering' – and like suffering, it lasts.

And this suffering spreads, from the individual, to those who care for them and about them, to their community, to the country as a whole. Dementia is, as one doctor said to me, 'profoundly disrespectful of patients, carers, health systems, social care . . . it doesn't fit into the structures we've created'. There can be no other illness that's so defined by its impact not just on those who live with it but on those around them. Its meanings are physiological, psychological, social, economic, political and philosophical. Its costs are unquantifiable – I don't mean the financial costs, though these are huge (the Alzheimer's Society estimates that, in the UK alone, the cost is £26 billion and, in the world, $818 billion – and steadily rising, set to teach $1 trillion by 2018 – more than the cost of cancer, stroke and heart disease combined), but the costs in human terms: the shame, confusion, fear, sorrow, guilt, loneliness. It provokes profound moral questions about the society in which we live, about the values we hold and about the meaning of life itself.

At the same time, we are the first generation to have really considered it mindfully. When I was a child, it was scarcely visible and rarely acknowledged. My grandfather on my mother's side of the family had dementia, as did my grandmother on my father's. Although I was aware of this, it was only in a muted way: they became like figures who had once been vivid in my life but were now being gradually rubbed out. I was perhaps embarrassed by them, these people who used to be figures of authority and now were so helpless, and I was also a bit queasy about the bodily nature of the disease, but I didn't think about what it was like for them or let myself imagine the tragedy that was being played out, sometimes in the form of a nasty farce. It was a stigma, a source of shame, fear and denial, and it went on behind closed doors. The D word.

We are aware of it now in a way that is radically different from twenty or thirty years ago and this awareness brings social, political and moral responsibility. Now we can see that which was previously hidden. In the seventies, there were about 300,000 people with dementia in the UK, spread thinly across the country. Today, there are three times that number. In twenty-five years' time, there will be something like 1.7 million. In the US, the incidence of death from Alzheimer's alone increased 55 per cent in the fifteen years between 1999 and 2014. Go into a hospital ward, even a general one, and several or most of the beds are occupied by people with dementia. Go into a residential home for the elderly. Look at the obituaries. (When I was thinking about this book, I began a list of all the well-known people who were dying with the illness, but I abandoned it: there were too many and they kept on coming; I couldn't keep up.) Read the news stories, the uplifting ones and the ones that make you want to howl in sorrow. I know scarcely anyone who doesn't have some kind of intimate connection to the disease. It's all around us, in our families and in our genes; perhaps in our own futures (approximately one out of six people over eighty get dementia, and the older the age the higher the chance; it's like there's a sniper in the garden). If it's not you or me, it's someone we love.

We can no longer just talk about 'them' – it's 'us' now, and how we face up to this challenge becomes a question of our collective humanity. For in an age where autonomy and agency are so highly valued, there are questions we urgently need to ask: what do we owe others and what do we owe ourselves? Who matters? Why do some people seem to matter less than others? Why do some people become ignored, invisible, neglected, abandoned? What is it to be human, and what is it to act in a human way? The word 'we' is used persistently and easily. It speaks of community, democracy, collaboration. It lays claim to a collective voice, as if we were, as the politicians like to say, all in this together. In the same boat – well, yes, but some people are in the first-class cabins with a sea view and cocktails at dinner, others are down in the hold, and still others are not seen at all. The light doesn't fall on them; we don't even realize they are on board with us. And quite a few have fallen into the cold water and they're drowning out there in the darkness, while the band plays on.

Those we do not see. Those we do not care about. Those we do not mourn. Those we neglect to the point of death . . . If my father had been an important man, I think he might have been treated differently at his time of greatest need – and of course, he *was* important, but only to those people who knew and loved him and whose lives were bound up with his. A sense of the preciousness of every life should be designed into a system, a society, so that we do not need to feel identification in order to rescue each other. We all have an obligation to each other – even to people we are hostile to – because the world is 'given to us in common', to share and to pass on. There is no *I* without a *you*, no *me* without *us*. We are at each other's mercy in the end, and we should have a passionate, unequivocal commitment to everyone, to anyone – honouring them not out of love but out of common humanity.

In the last few years, I have been thinking a great deal about the meaning of rules and of boundaries: the walls of institutions on which rules – *thou shalt not* – are posted; the fences around gardens, the doors (that can be shut fast or open), the borders (that are often more porous than I understood), the minds (that are also embodied); the bodies (that both contain us and yet expose us to the world), the *I* and the *we*, the *us* and the *them*, self and other. How much are we connected to each other and how much are we separated? How far are we private, discrete people and how far part of a public, communal life? How much can we – should we – rely on others and be relied on in our turn? What are our responsibilities to the world in which we live, and then what are our responsibilities to our self?

As a mother, I sometimes have difficulty in knowing where my children end and I begin (even though they are all adults now and I really should have learned). I can feel to myself too much like an open wound and I don't know how to say no. At

7

the same time, I'm a lifelong feminist who believes whole-heartedly in the right to have a life that belongs, at least in part, to oneself. Attachment and responsibility and, above all, love, continually threaten self-belonging. The claustrophobia I can sometimes feel at my responsibilities is a fear of self-loss. We all need boundaries to possess a self, and we all need to breach those boundaries in order to live in a world of relation-ships and connections – for what other world is there? It's not a balancing act, quivering and tense on a tightrope hung between two opposing imperatives, but a continuing flux: advancing and retreating; giving and withholding, reaching out into the world and retreating back from it.

Dementia undoes this delicate and endless negotiation with the world, this tidal shift of reciprocity. Bit by bit, those living with it become helpless, at the mercy of others and reliant on the kindness of people who are close to them and of strangers. It is hardly bearable to think how lonely and beyond reach they must sometimes feel. A few weeks ago, I was in a care home with Sean (my husband and writing partner), visiting one of his relatives who has dementia. As we were leaving, an old woman stumbled towards us; she was wearing a cheery red cardigan and beads and her shoulder-length hair was white; on her face was a look of anguish. I stopped and she grasped my hands and her body bent in grief. 'Hymns of comfort,' she said. 'Hymns of comfort.' I looked around for someone to help her. I told her they were coming soon. 'No one is coming,' she said. 'No one is here. Hymns of comfort.' A member of staff arrived and took the buckled figure from me. She said – as if this made it all right – that the woman was always behaving like this, and she led her away. 'Hymns of comfort.' What should I have done? What are we doing?

To explore dementia's meaning and its excruciating losses is to think about how far we as a society and as individuals are responsible for the suffering of others: what we owe each other, what we care about, what matters in this world we all share. *Who* matters.

At the word 'dementia', many people jump-cut forward to the imagined end. They see themselves or the person they love stripped of all memory and capacity, lying befuddled in a bed; they see themselves as aged babies (although the comparison between old people at the end of their life with small children is cruelly inappropriate), animals, vegetables, *objects* that other people handle or neglect. Many people emphatically state their determination to end their life well before they get to this end; some people do so. Mary Warnock famously argued for a licence to 'put people down', and while this sounds harsh and was controversial, there is an argument that we put animals down when their life has become one of intolerable suffering but we do not extend the same kindness to humans who have to endure beyond the limits of endurance. What we wouldn't do to a dog we do to ourselves.

But there are many stages in dementia, as there are in grief— although as with grief these stages are rarely clear and steady. The diagnosis is not a sentence but the start of a process that can take years, even decades, and that can contain hope and kindness and adventure as well as fear and sorrow and heart-wrenching loss.

This book is a journey through those stages of loss, from the first vague signs of the illness through to advanced, end-of-life dementia, which at its most radical can seem like a ferocious de-creation of the self and an apocalypse of meaning. It asks what dementia means, both for the person who lives with the condition and for those who love them. It looks at both the kindest and the most inhumane forms of professional intervention, and asks how far professionals can 'care' for those we care about and how much individuals and families must shoulder a burden whose weight can – and often does – crush lives. It explores dementia from the outside and – as far as it is possible – from the inside as well. It looks at the new and unsettling art that is being made about dementia – which is, I believe, a form of emotional modernism and which can help us imagine what is unimaginable, to find a language for that which is essentially wordless, taking us up to the threshold of darkness. It looks at the grief that is felt on the journey into darkness, both by the person with an illness that brings such desolation and also by those who care for them. And it looks at the aftermath of a life: at death, mourning and the kindness of an ending. It contains the stories of nurses, doctors, scientists, therapists, philosophers, artists – but above all, of people who are living with this disease and those who are accompanying them, bearing the unbearable, becoming the gatekeeper, the memory and the voice. Dementia calls forth what Atul Gawande calls 'the endurance of the soul'.

My guide has been my father, vigorous at first and then frail, sometimes disappearing from view. He had also been my ghost. Always my ghost.

In the early stages – which are perhaps the ones that hold the most agony for the affected individual, or at least I hope so; I hope forgetfulness brings a form of relief – people with dementia can express their feelings. Later, it becomes more and more difficult for them to do so, until at last it is barely possible. What must it be like? Quite often I wake in the small hours of the morning, before light has come, and for a terrifying moment I can't remember where I am or even who I am. An appalling blank that is followed by a scorching fear. Does this give a glimpse into what it feels like? Or that sense of humiliating befuddlement when one has lost track of everything and is slack and stranded in a muddle of thoughts, no traction and no grip on the world, an object not a subject: is that it?

A few months ago, I was cycling along a canal in the middle of the night; it was very dark and dislocating and eerie. There was duckweed on the water, so the water looked like solid ground while the solid ground wavered and shifted under the thin beam from my bike lamp. Bats like dark rags just above me; voices suddenly heard in the distance and then silence. I was unsafe. Unsafe in myself, small and unstable and swilling with dread. I felt, with a ghastly lurch, that perhaps this too was what someone might feel in the early stages of dementia: everything that was once certain now losing its shape, things looming out of the gloom. But I don't know, of course. The mind is infinitely mysterious. And if it is hard to imagine the earlier stages, when the person is still articulate, how much harder to understand what it is like to have advanced dementia, a condition beyond language. There's an existential loneliness and even despair about it: to become one's own ghost.

For how does the *I* observe the *I* that is going, and how can language capture its own disintegration? Talking with people living with dementia, there can be eloquent gaps and slippages in their descriptions of what they are experiencing. When we talk *about* them – and inevitably, most of the accounts of advanced dementia are external – we turn to metaphor, using language to grope for what lies beyond words. From Dante's image of a ship lowering its sails as it enters harbour, to comparisons with a deck of cards reshuffled, we try to find ways of comprehending the incomprehensible de-creation of the self. I know that I have variously described my father as a great ship untethered and slipping out to sea, a town whose lights are going out one by one, a bombed city, an ice floe breaking up and becoming smaller and smaller until there is no place left to stand. A friend described it as a manuscript ripped into tiny shreds; another as a precious glass, smashed. It's striking how often the image of a ship is used – a boat going into the mist; 'a sailing vessel that is becalmed. And then suddenly there is a breeze. I am sailing again. Then the world has a hold on me again.'

The notion of being at sea conjures both the terror and the mystery; there's a solemnity and a dignity in this metaphor that sails grandly and kindly over the nasty horrors of the deep. In his harrowing meditation on his mother's early and cruel dementia, *Stammered Songbook*, the Belgian writer Erwin Mortier struggles to make meaning and give shape to what is meaningless and shapeless. He conjures up a disease that is not grand but vicious and ratty, sneaking underground, eating away at wires with its sharp yellow teeth – it wrings his mother out 'like a floorcloth' and slings her in a corner. It's a stagnant fen, a tide going out. His mother is a buckled cage with a mechanical songbird rusting away inside, an hourglass of skin and bone, a house that's slowly collapsing, grammatical ruin, an old valve radio, an owl chick somewhere in the tangle of collapsed beams; one great vanishing point.

Metaphors used about dementia evoke disappearance and dissolution (the sea, the mist, the lowering of the sails), but also corrosion, fracture, queasy slippage and a sinister mutation of the self. They are an attempt to give meaning and shape to what resists both, making a fragile bridge between the known and the unknowable and at the same time signalling the impossibility of the task. The ocean becomes the swamp; the house becomes its basement. Terror lurches into horror, horror is suddenly brightened by hope, a shaft of light through wreckage. Language strains to accommodate a condition that is profoundly connected to the failure of language and the connection of the self to the world. Words fail.

But words are not the only way of speaking. On my desk, I have images of the self-portraits by the London-based German-American artist William Utermohlen. I never met him but I have spent many hours talking to his widow, Patricia Utermohlen, and I often return to his paintings to remind myself of the special terror of dementia. Utermohlen was formally diagnosed with Alzheimer's in 1995 when he was sixty-one, although the hints of his illness may be seen in his 'Conversation Pieces' of the early nineties. Unsparingly, he looked at himself and painted himself even as he lost the sense of himself. His self-portraits over the next five years give a sense of excruciating instability, haunting self-loss. In the first, he is recognizably himself, although his thin face has a watchful expression (he was, Patricia tells me, an anxious and disappointed man). But quickly the perspectives flatten, the spatial sense is lost. He is both inside the world of self-loss and observing it. He is inscribing the dementia on to the canvas. The neuropsychologist Professor Seb Crust, who was one of his doctors, remembers how, when they met, Utermohlen skilfully made a sketch, and yet in it both arms were coming out of one shoulder. At the same time the portraits give a unique narrative of the artist's subjective experience, in which the order and sensory richness of the first give way to a disquieting strangeness, a sensory dislocation in which walls tip, perspectives are destabilized, the table lifts up, objects float and an ill wind blows through the dismantled room in which the artist sits and watches what he is becoming – or unbecoming. Things are torn, broken, crushed, dissolved and lost. The space empties and at last the painter is alone in a void. The face, the self, recedes and disappears in shadows. In the final portrait he is simply a scribbled death-head.

Seen individually, Utermohlen self-portraits are profoundly sad. Seen as a series, they are terrifying in their portrayal of loss over time, suffering over time, the gradual, inevitable stripping away of all that holds him together in the shape of a man. And yet for several years of living with Alzheimer's, William Utermohlen was at home with his wife and his paintings; he saw friends and remained in the rich flow of life. Above all, he continued to express himself, putting his mark on the canvas, saying, *I am here*. To be human is to have a voice – and by *voice* I mean that which connects our inner and outer worlds, the delicate and miraculous web of communications that ensures we live in community with others, not in solitary confinement with ourselves. There are many different ways to have a voice and to reach out into the world.

Even when memory is gone, language is splintered and lost, recognition has crumbled, and the notion of a self is hard to hold on to, there are ways to find the human being trapped in the wreckage, to hear them and to acknowledge that they are still humans, precious, and one of us.

One of my friends died when he was fifty, after a decade of living with a brain tumour. Ten years later, I still dream about him quite often. He's my night visitor and it's always a joy to see him; I remember how I've missed him. In several recent dreams, we have been jumping on a trampoline together. Sometimes he doesn't realize that he's dead but I do and we talk about this. Sometimes I believe he has returned; his deadness is a mistake, a dream itself, or it is out of bounds back there in the waking world. But as far as I know, I've never once dreamed of my father. He never visits me. Perhaps this is because I don't properly believe that he has died. Part of me feels that I can have a second chance and can do it all better this time, see what's happening to him more swiftly and make it unhappen, turn back the clock that ticked him to his end. 'Hello, Nic,' he'll say, and hold out his hand.

I want to remember my father as he was before his illness, and I do – but the image that most often flashes up in me and takes me unawares is of him in his final months, when I am looking at him through the window, lying propped up on his hospital bed, staring out at the garden he had made and loved. Gone and still here; part of life and banished from it. Shortly after my father died, I launched a campaign with a friend that fights for more compassionate hospital care for those with dementia. Of course, I know that in part I'm trying save my father, who's beyond rescue. So too, in writing this book, I realize that secretly I 'write partly to make a confession', or as the French philosopher Jacques Derrida has it: as soon as you write you are asking for forgiveness.

1. *Facing Up*

'I am! yet what I am none cares or knows.'

Sean and I have a house in a comfortable area of north London, where we write our psychological thrillers under the name Nicci French. The Victorian terraced buildings on the tree-lined street are attractive, with well-tended gardens and geraniums in window-boxes. There's a small green where people throw sticks for their dogs, a playground. There's a primary school; each weekday morning little children cluster outside its gates, a babble of bright voices. There are restaurants, cafés and shops a few minutes away. And at the far end of the road stands a huge prison, its high walls topped with barbed wire; at its rear are unmarked graves where executed prisoners used to be buried. I sometimes see windowless vans driving in through the gates, or out of them, and quite often at night there are helicopters hovering like giant chirring insects above it, spotlights swinging through darkness. People say they've spotted drones around the building as well, dropping drugs or mobile phones. But I can't see in; I've never glimpsed any of the people who are incarcerated there; never heard their voices.

Bad things, terrible things, go on inside this prison, where more than 1,200 men live in overcrowded, squalid, inhumane conditions. Twelve-foot by eight-foot cells built for a single occupant often hold two men, with a badly screened toilet just a few feet from where they eat and sleep. The toilets are often blocked; the sewage leaks; there is rubbish on the floors; cockroaches have a field day; the budget for their meals is not much more than £1.50 a day, like swill for pigs. Drugs are pervasive, especially the new 'zombie' drug Spice, which induces a semi-comatose state, enabling the inmates to better endure their time. Gangs are in control. There's bullying and violence and suicide and a climate of misery and fear. But we outside go on with our comfortable lives, not wanting to think about this institution right next door. These men are out of sight, out of mind, shut away from the world and stripped of their basic rights as humans. Indeed, many people believe that prisoners have forfeited their human rights; they deserve punishment, are not owed anything. In a culture of credits and debits, they are paying their dues. So it's easy to forget about them: not one of us, after all.

We often feel and act because of a sense of identification: a person is like us or represents a world we are familiar with or aspire to. In some way or other, they feel *near* to us, intimate, and if they are in danger we have a fierce rescue impulse. Some people are injured, or abused, or go missing, and we care, with a surge of empathy. Some people go missing and we're indifferent. Some go missing and we don't even know.

At the end of 1995 and into the start of 1996 I covered the long, grim trial of Rosemary West for the *Observer*. Frederick and Rosemary West had been an apparently ordinary provincial couple living with their children, getting on with their neighbours, drinking mugs of tea and cooking Sunday roasts, who over a span of sixteen years sexually abused and murdered their own children, and tortured and killed other young women. They were serial killers who treated their victims like living sex aids before burying them in their garden. Fred West killed himself while in prison, so only his wife stood in the dock, in a trial that gripped the country and still has resonance today. For several weeks during that winter, a window was half opened on to a world most of us had never imagined existed, a world of obscenity, degradation and unravelled violence. It was as if a scene from Hieronymous Bosch had been played out over many years in a small terraced house in Gloucester that was abattoir, brothel and Sadeian torture chamber all at once. By the end of the trial, when Rosemary West was convicted of ten counts of murder and given life imprisonment, I felt I had been poisoned and needed to somehow cleanse myself.

But alongside the feeling of horror and foulness – a world turned upside down – there was a less garish but more enduring sense of loss that changed the stories I wanted to write as a journalist and even the way I thought about the world. Several of the young women who got sucked into the black hole of 25 Cromwell Street over the years had disappeared with barely a ripple; some were never reported missing. The Wests usually chose people who were vulnerable and powerless, who had been in care, who were unemployed or rootless and did not belong to a community. They had no safety nets. When these women and girls went missing, they were not missed. There was no frantic search, no nationwide grief, no lament. They were invisible people and when they disappeared they remained invisible and largely unmourned. Only when their bodies were found many years later did they briefly claim our attention.

Some months after the trial ended, I spent several weeks with London prostitutes, sitting in dimly lit and overheated rooms hearing about their lives, stepping out when clients arrived. They were all young, some still teenagers; most of them had been physically or sexually abused; all but one was a crack addict; almost all had been in care of one kind or another – and heartbreakingly, what several said they most wanted to do if they got a chance was to be a foster parent themselves, rescuing kids like themselves; rescuing their younger selves. The street they worked was a stone's throw from where I live now. It's since been transformed into an area of corporate cool, but then it was run-down and surrounded by wastelands where the women took their clients if they weren't lucky enough to have a room. Why hadn't I noticed them before?

We each live in a tiny pool of light, and around us lies the darkness of our un-seeing. We see what we look for and what we look at. There is an experiment first conducted nearly two decades ago and repeated in various forms since that demonstrates this 'inattentional blindness': people are shown a video and asked to keep a silent count of how many times basketball players, three dressed in white and three in black, pass a ball between each other. After about thirty seconds, a woman in a gorilla suit enters the rooms, faces the camera and thumps her chest, then walks away. See this video knowingly and it's dumbfounding that anyone could fail to notice her. But half the viewers miss her: they are busy concentrating on the players and they aren't looking for her, and so she is invisible.

(I have my own version of this story. One summer holiday, my daughter, aged about three, her elder brother and her cousin were sitting on a jetty, fishing with their makeshift rods. She was between the two of them, and all of a sudden she tipped forward and neatly plopped into the lake. The two boys continued fishing; they only reacted when a fully clothed adult charged past them and jumped into the water.)

We are all trapped by the limits of our mind. It's not possible to see the world we live in, only minute, shuttered portions of it where the beam of our attention falls. When I was a teenager, I noticed other teenagers. Pregnant, I suddenly saw all the pregnant women; then the babies; and then the world was full of small children and their exhausted parents; full of single mothers . . . Now I see countless people who are frail and scared – but that's only because I saw my father so frail and so scared.

We can't see everything, but perhaps we can learn to be more aware of just how blind we are and make some kind of amends. A few years ago, when I was working on a novel called *Missing Persons*, I spent weeks wandering around London, suddenly seeing what had always been there: the figures under the arches, the people huddled in doorways, in Underground stations, on benches, in makeshift tents, pushing supermarket trolleys filled with plastic bags of tatty possessions, holding out cardboard signs saying 'Help Me', old beyond their years, faces burnt by sun and wind, matted hair, thick beards, trying to meet the eyes of those who pass them – who are trying very hard not to meet their eyes, who are making a wide circle to avoid them. Walking through a grim underpass in a big city, I see fliers posted on columns: 'When did you last see a homeless person?' And further on, the response: 'The more you see, the less you see.' The homeless and the dispossessed, who have fallen through every safety net, remind us of what happens when luck fails. Best not to look: not one of us, after all.

Every life is precious: so easy to think and to say, much harder to feel and act upon. What if the person who suffers is different? What if they come from far away, in rickety boats? What if they are lying in a doorway in a rank sleeping bag with a can of white cider in their hand and an ugly, loyal dog beside them?

And what if they are old, forgetful, decrepit, adrift and seem like creatures from a world we don't want to think about? For many decades, those living with dementia have also been missing people in our society. Sometimes they have withdrawn (or have been withdrawn) from the public sphere and are out of sight, in hospitals, in care homes, behind closed doors. Sometimes they are more existentially invisible. Because they are helpless, at the mercy of others, a kind of erasure of social meaning turns them into forlorn and ghostly figures. They are there but not really there, not part of the thick flow of life. The light does not fall on them.

I remember being in a restaurant when my father was in the early stages of his great decline, and he was having difficulty with his order, on a loop of indecision. The young waitress was smirking and rolling her eyes at us, as if we were in on the great joke. I followed her when she left the table and gave her a dressing-down; she looked so bewildered and upset that I was ashamed of myself. She wasn't cruel; she just didn't know, didn't understand. She thought she was in a different kind of play – a light-hearted farce, not a tragic one.

And I've lost count of the times that I've witnessed people being impatient, maybe a bit contemptuous, of men and women in public spaces who are old and confused and slowing things up (of the times I've been like this myself). Or the occasions that I've witnessed good, hard-working doctors and nurses talking about and across their frail, confused patients rather than to them; snapping on plastic gloves before they touch them, without explanation, as if their bodies were contaminated objects; looking at computer screens rather than at the vulnerable and often anxious person who's in an unfamiliar situation and needs their help; just seeming a bit in a hurry or a bit indifferent, other things on their mind. I will always be grateful to one of my father's doctors, a melancholy and exhausted-looking man from Eastern Europe whose manner was invariably one of tender respect. I've no idea what he was like as a clinician – but my father was at a point in his life when he no longer needed a gifted clinician but a sympathetic human being who would ask his permission to sit on the bed and take his hand, talk to him deferentially, address him formally by his title (Doctor), recognize that, for all his losses, he remained a subject, an *I*.

As with so many other groups of the forgotten, it is easier to ignore those living with dementia if they are subtly dehumanized, made *less*. It is built into the way we talk about them, the stock phrases we use without stopping to consider their implications: they are not the person they used to be, we say; they are not all there and they are no longer themselves. They are shadows of themselves. As the loss deepens, the language becomes starker: we say that they are gone, minds become sieves. We say that they have lost their mind (where is it, then?), or are out of their mind (where are they, then?). And perhaps we say that they are mindless: the living dead.

Not one of us.

We are all diminished if we think like this.

Several years ago, one of my daughters fell off a horse and was knocked unconscious. She was taken by ambulance to the nearby hospital, where she was kept in overnight because not only could she not remember the accident, nor the weeks preceding it, neither could she make new memories. She was on a loop: every time we told her what had happened, she would express surprise in identical words, with identical intonations, with the exact same expression of comic disbelief – and then a few minutes later ask for an explanation again. The ward was a general orthopaedic one, but except for my daughter and another woman who was calmly reading a book, her glasses balanced on the end of her nose, every other patient was old and had dementia. My daughter's condition in some ways mimicked theirs – she was unable to remember – but she was going to recover her memories; they were not.

Since then, I've visited many hospitals and become more used to what they are like, but at the time I was very shocked, and also scared to be leaving my daughter there. The air felt thick with distress, helplessness and fear. Several of the women were lying slack and unresponsive, mouths open; they looked sick and absent from the world. One woman was writhing on her bed and screaming the same words over and over: 'No, no, please don't. Teacher, don't.' She had her hands on her stomach: 'It's down there,' she cried. I imagine she was perhaps reliving some kind of trauma: while most memories had been washed away, this ugly one remained, repeated, a nightmare she couldn't wake up from because she *was* awake and buried in herself. It looked like a kind of fresh hell to me. The nurses were extraordinarily patient and respectful, but there was no way that they could respond to everyone, and probably they had become used to it. In a ward of people with dementia, this amount of distress and chaos was normal, like a kind of background noise.

Not long ago, I visited a ward where one of the patients was in a pitiful state. She could barely speak but she knew she wanted to go home; had to go home. She kept trying to get out of bed, to escape back to where she felt safe and cherished, which was probably somewhere long ago. A young doctor, stopping by on her ward round, explained why they were not going to be able to let her leave, however much she wanted to; it was for her own good. The woman wept; her face was wet with tears and she could not be comforted.

Or another ward at another time: a woman lay immobile,

only her bony hands fluttering; so thin her frame barely disturbed the sheets. On the table next to her was a photograph in which a radiant girl from the distant past stands on a beach, ankle deep in the waves, holding the hand of a man and smiling. It was painfully hard to reconcile these two selves – the woman in the bed and the one on the beach, the one in love with the future before her and the other approaching death.

Or in a care home visiting the mother of a friend, where a tall, skinny, snaggle-toothed woman came up to me and gripped my hand hard, clearly upset and trying to tell me something, her eyes glittering with the need to communicate. But I couldn't make out a syllable; she was talking in nobody's language. Words that weren't words poured from her. Nobody could understand her: there's loneliness.

The culture around dementia is changing; the illness that used to be hidden away is now recognized and talked about, the subject of political initiatives, international research, global campaigns. No country and no community can escape the disease and almost every country and community has found ways of ameliorating the lives of those who live with it. There are hundreds and thousands of charities throughout the world, some huge and far-reaching like the Alzheimer's Society, with a presence in dozens of countries, and some small and specific, like the tiny, local one I am patron of, the Creative Dementia Arts Network, which focuses on the power of creative arts in dementia.

There are imaginative new ways of approaching the illness. In countries including the Netherlands and Denmark there are dementia villages, places that enable their residents to preserve their sense of autonomy. In the US, the collaborative Dementia Friendly Initiative has been set up to foster nationwide awareness and dementia-friendliness. In Japan – whose ageing population means that about 5 million people live with dementia, a figure set to rise to 7 million by 2025 – there are a host of recent devices to monitor and care for those who are frail and confused (a teapot sensor, for instance, that transmits an alert to a family member if tea hasn't been made for some time; a sticker with a QR code in case that person is lost, for lostness is an increasing problem; robots that will fetch food or provide comfort).

In Denmark, most municipalities have set up activity centres for the old to reduce the risk of inactivity. In Dresden, a nursing home has re-created an entire historical era (of communist East Germany) in order to reactivate memories and bring vitality to the lives of their elderly residents. In the UK (as in many other countries), there's dementia training in hospitals and out of them, supermarkets where all the staff wear dementia-friendly badges, whole towns that are aiming to be 'dementia friendly'. There are partnerships between nurseries and old people's homes; collaborations between residential homes and schools; exchange programmes in which university students live rent free in a nursing home in return for a set number of hours a month acting as neighbours to the often isolated residents; intergenerational housing developments . . .

And there seem to be conferences for every day of the year at which people from all over the world come together to pool knowledge and share ideas. We know the figures, the scarifying percentages, the graphs with lines that rise like a jagged cliff, up and away into oblivion. Hollywood films, bestselling memoirs, documentaries, plays, sobering headlines, optimistic ones. The word 'dementia' has almost become a prefix. When I went to the 2017 UK Dementia Congress, held at a racecourse, the vast hall was full of stands advertising dementia mattresses, dementia decorations (images of flowing water and bright flowers), dementia clocks, publications, projects, food, care homes, hoists . . . It seems ridiculous to say that people with dementia are like missing persons.

And yet: old men wandering down the corridors with their pyjamas round their ankles. Old women weeping and unconsoled. People lashing out at doctors and nurses. Patients called 'bed-blockers' or, in the US, 'GOMERs' (Get Out of My Emergency Room), and the dedicated healthcare staff doing their best not to see them as objects, burdens, statistics and problems, so that someone crying out, 'Help me! Help Me!' is just irritating, their words of agony mere verbal tics.

Each year, news stories reveal the neglect and abuse that goes on behind closed doors – because to be a professional carer is a woefully undervalued and underpaid occupation, and if someone can't remember they can't tell tales; and because as a culture we have infantilized and even dehumanized the old, frail and cognitively impaired.

Dementia can bring soul-sickness and despair. In April of 2017, a ninety-five-year-old man was spared a prison sentence for trying to bludgeon his beloved eighty-eight-year-old wife ('the most beautiful woman in the world') to death with a lump hammer and a ceramic pan after she repeatedly begged him to kill her. She had 'fragile' mental health and he was her carer, resolutely refusing assistance from social services. She wanted him to kill her before she had to go into hospital or a home, 'And I haven't managed to,' he said to the police officers who came to their home, 'and now I have just increased her suffering . . . I would happily be a murderer. Please tell me I killed her.'

To want to die rather than be dependent and helpless, in a home away from a marriage of sixty-five years; to try to kill the person you love the most because their future seems mere torment: what does this say about our culture? If a person ceases to be a moral agent, in control of their lives, if they cease to have self-consciousness and rationality, a narrative sense of themselves, does that mean that they are less of a person and their life less valuable? What is it to be alive, after all? Dementia is one of those disorders that 'seriously jeopardizes the faculties we ordinarily define as uniquely human: memory, personality, recognition, awareness, the capacity to love, even a sense of hope. The brain, the mind, the spirit, and the will . . . which constitute the central locus of humanity, are affected.' What does it mean for individuals to live 'under conditions that place them outside the usual criteria used to describe humanness'?

In her scorching memoir, *Keeper*, about the two years she lived with her mother-in-law and her rapidly worsening Alzheimer's disease, Andrea Gillies asks, 'What it is that dementia takes away?' And she answers herself: 'Everything; every last thing we reassure ourselves that nothing could take away from us.' It's the dementia abyss, into which meaning is sucked.

The day after her riding accident, we collected our daughter from hospital. Her ability to form new memories was returning, but she had no memory of the night she had spent among all the women who had been calling out for help, shouting, swearing, crying. And I too soon forgot about that shadowy world of distress and loss. I closed the door on it, for a while.

2. Getting Older

'Oldness has come . . . the heart is forgetful'

If you are lucky enough for life to take its expected course, then 'you will be old for longer than you were ever young'.

The world's population is ageing. According to a UN report, the number of people over sixty is projected to grow by 56 per cent between 2015 and 2030, from 901 million to 1.4 billion; by 2050, the global population of older people is projected to be double the size it was in 2015, reaching 2.1 billion. The global number of people over eighty – the so-called 'oldest-old' – is growing even faster overall: in 2015, there were 125 million people over eighty; in 2050, it is projected there will be 434 million. Crucially, the number of older people is growing faster than the numbers of people in any other age group: in other words, the share of older people in the total population is swiftly increasing. By 2050, one in five people will be over sixty; in high-income countries, where the pace of population ageing is rapid, the percentage is already much higher than this (33 per cent in Japan, for instance). In the UK (where life expectancy has actually fallen in the last three years), there were just fewer than 15,000 centenarians in 2016, while life expectancy for a baby boy was 79.2 years, and for a baby girl 82.9 years. It used to be that a man or woman could expect a handful of years after they retired; now it's maybe fifteen or twenty, almost a quarter of an average life span. There's an argument that old age should be redefined, in favour of 'prospective age', when the remaining life expectancy falls below fifteen years. Sixty (speaking as someone who nearly is) doesn't have the same meaning it used to have; seventy barely counts as old.

But although life expectancy is so much higher and old age has become a hefty slice in the pie chart of our lives however it is measured, it doesn't seem that we've got used to it, or welcomed it, or found a way to accommodate the shape of our lives to it. It's like the material left over at the end that we – individually and as a society – don't know what to do with. In the US, poverty among pensioners stands at over 20 per cent (in Australia it is around a startling 35 per cent) and many Americans live in fear of retiring poor. In the UK, about 1.7 million pensioners are living in poverty, and a quarter of older households live in non-decent housing. What's more, according to a recent survey, more than three quarters of old people feel lonely; two fifths of those over seventy-five say that television is their main company.

For some (those who have money and health, family and friends, good fortune), old age can be a time of great happiness. For others, it is scary and desolating, a bitter end to a long life. How do we fund the extra years? How do we better care for those who are old and have health problems? How do we rebalance society so that everyone – the young, the middle-aged, the elderly, the very old – can have a purpose and can flourish? And how long will it take before being old is not in some strange way a bit humiliating, a bit of a failure, something of a disgrace?

Several years ago I was in a large department store, running late, looking for things I couldn't find, hot and feeling a bit frazzled and itchy and out of sorts. As I was hastening along an aisle, a woman came hastening towards me. She was quite a bit older than I was, scrawny, and looked distressed and in a state of substantial disarray. As I drew closer I saw her shirt was wrongly buttoned. I put up a hand to prevent her bumping into me, and she put up a hand as well, smiling anxiously back at me. I stopped. She stopped. We stared at each other with a kind of pity. And with a sudden rush of mortification, I understood that she was me. I was looking at myself in a mirror. Usually, we prepare ourselves for our reflection. Here, I was caught unawares and my self-image shattered and lay in pieces around me. I stood face to face with the self that others see.

Was I that tired and shambolic? Was I that *old*? That woman in the mirror wasn't me. It never is.

That moment comes back to me when I'm on an Underground train. It is morning and crowded, with no spare seats. I stand in the aisle, put in my earplugs, turn on my music, tune out.

Then all of a sudden a polite young man is rising from his seat. He gestures to me, offering his place.

I stare at him wildly. I look around at the other passengers who are standing – surely lots of them are older than me. That woman with grey hair and a creased face: she must be a decade ahead of me. Perhaps he means her. But no, it's me he is making way for.

I shake my head and thank him but tell him I am getting off at the next station – which I wasn't, but of course then have to, hot-faced with the sense of my own absurdity. When the next train arrives it too is crowded so I stand next to the door, my face averted so no one can see me and kindly offer me their seat.

I speak to a friend of my age about the experience (swapping those consoling tales of middle-age humiliations) and she says yes, oh my god yes, she was offered a seat recently and was so agitated that she sat plump down on it and burst into tears. Like me, she insisted that there were lots of other people standing who were years – no, decades – older than her.

They probably weren't older than her, just as the woman with grey hair in my carriage probably wasn't older than me. But we often fail to see ourselves as middle-aged, though we know we are; or old, though we know we are. (Simone de Beauvoir observed in *Old Age* that the old tend to say 'them' rather than 'us'.) The person in the mirror is a shock, rising towards us in the morning wearing the face of someone we never thought to become, gazing at us in horror from a future that has arrived before we are ready for it. Why did I so mind that a courteous stranger saw me as an older woman? I am, after all. What is it about getting older that I resist or don't entirely believe? I don't try to look younger than I am. I don't disguise my wrinkles (though I do buy anti-ageing cream, knowing it doesn't work). Most of the time, I like it that my face is marked by experience, like a map of my life. (Or in part I do, I say I do, I want to. Nevertheless, there are days when I scrutinize myself in the mirror, the pouches under the eyes, the brackets around the mouth and the lines above it, like I've been stitched up; the chipped tooth, the thinning skin that's lost its elasticity, and feel a bit anxious and dismayed.) I would never have cosmetic surgery. I would never conceal my age, although on websites, scrolling down through the years until I get to 1958, I always feel a slight surprise at the sight of how much time I've already gone through. I've long ago got used to the fact that my children now walk faster than me, swim faster, bike faster, think faster . . . As I grow older, I often experience invisibility as a gift, not an insult. Yet when a young man stands up for me, when I meet myself in a mirror, it still seems like a category error.

Recently, at a book-signing in the Netherlands, two Dutch men of about my age came up to me. They gave me a slim, hard-backed notebook and, smiling, watched me as I opened it. It was full of photos of the three of us thirty-nine years ago: sitting on a train, sailing a little dinghy on a cold and windy day, changing the tyre on a car while roaring with laughter. In one, we are in a crowd of people celebrating the end of a friend's finals at university. I was twenty then. I look rather drunk, very carefree and happy, very young, clutching a bottle of champagne. I stood in the bookshop staring at these pictures of the past, at these two strangers who turned out to be long-lost friends, and could barely speak for the complicated mix of emotions that winded me: amazement and gladness and sadness and disbelief that we had become these middle-aged, creased creatures with marriages and children and jobs and cars and houses. The past at that moment seemed more powerful and real than the present.

We suffer from 'temporal vertigo', absorbing all the ages we have ever been. That old woman I saw lying in a hospital bed beside the photograph of herself joyful on a beach long ago housed both the old and young self and everything in between. We identify ourselves as young, because in one sense we still are. The older, current self is a newcomer, still something of a stranger, who we have to live with but who we don't feel entirely comfortable with and may sometimes be distressed by. The heart takes time to catch up with a change that feels like a cinematic jump-cut. You're young and starting out, eager and full of hope – and all of a sudden, you're middle-aged: a crumpled, pouchy face gazes in startled outrage from the mirror. It is easy to know what it is to be young for everyone has been and still is, somewhere inside, and it is hard for the young (and even for the old) to imagine being old, for we see the old at a distance, through the wrong end of a telescope. Hard and disturbing and even appalling. That will never be me.

I think back a year or so, talking to my agent (about the idea for this book, in fact). We were sitting in her room, me on a sofa that felt slightly too low and too soft, so I was cast backwards, already a bit collapsed. It was hot; I was hot (menopausally so, with the raging urge to take most of my clothes off, particularly my shoes and socks, which I didn't). I was trying to find something in my bike pannier that I had printed out, but the pannier was large and full of bits and pieces, and anyway I couldn't locate my glasses, which were actually dangling around my neck; when I found them and tried to put them on, they got tangled with my bike keys that I hang around me with a ribbon like I'm my own hook, and also with my necklace. I felt encumbered, incompetent, shabby, graceless. I looked up and saw my agent, young and smooth-faced, her eyes kind, looking at me as I fumbled.

Twenty or so years before that, I was at a launch party for the re-publication of J. G. Links's magisterial guide to Venice, first published in 1973; Links was dead by then, but his widow, Mary Lutyens, was there. I knew a bit about her: she was a theosophist and sometime mystic – the biographer of Krishnamurti, admirer of Gandhi and fierce critic of the Raj – a vegetarian, a believer in tolerance, a traveller, a novelist, a scholar of art history and a distinguished biographer. She was clever, free-spirited, beautiful and full of curiosity. At this party, she must have been about eighty-eight years old, her wonderful face a mosaic of wrinkles. She was in a wheelchair, and the party flowed around her, like a river around a stone. Guests had to bend down to speak to her. They talked loudly (I don't know if she was deaf; nor I think did they) and slowly, separating out each word as if she had trouble understanding things now, or as if they did not share a common language. I remember seeing the expression on her face, which was one of magnificent fury.

At about the same time as this, I interviewed P. L. Travers (who wrote the great *Mary Poppins* books) for the *Observer* newspaper. She was clearly near the end of her life. Her face was ravaged by time. She could no longer walk (she told me her aim was to be able to reach the first lamp post on her road, but I think she never managed this) and she had trouble speaking; every word was an effort and had a cost and a value. I had never met anyone as old as she was: she seemed to me then to have come from a different age, a relic of past glories, and I regarded her with a kind of awe. She knew that she would soon die and, with painful slowness, she told me something of her life and her philosophy – although she was a private woman, fierce and proud and solitary, and when I left her I felt that I had barely scratched the surface of her mystery. Late that night, she rang me and in her ancient, halting, rumbling voice told me that she wept her secrets into her pillow every night; no one would ever know her soul. Shortly after this encounter I heard that she had died. I've never forgotten her: she gave me a glimpse into the uncanny depths of the human mind and showed me – I shouldn't have needed showing, but I did – that in age people become *more*. They gather up all their selves. In that battered, sore body of hers, the body that she couldn't haul to the first lamp post up the road, in that impenetrable mind, she held the hidden richness of her past.

My mother is old and nearly blind, bashed about by multiple strokes, but indomitable and so full of spirit you can warm yourself by standing near her. Sometimes when I am with her people will pat her hand call her 'dear' and 'sweetheart', as though she were a child again. And when my father was lying in his bed in the downstairs room I found myself calling him 'sweetheart', calling him 'poppet' and 'darling', as if he were a baby and I his crooning mother. My father, who was so modest and so dignified.

(Raymond Tallis – the philosopher, poet, novelist, cultural critic, humanist, patron of Dignity in Dying, retired medical physician specializing in geriatrics and all-round extraordinary person – tells me that if anyone ever calls him 'poppet', he will be hard-pressed not to 'top them'. A keenly intelligent man, he is also humane; he thinks feelingly. When he was still practising as a doctor in Manchester, he insisted that his staff give patients their proper name, Mrs or Mr or Ms or Dr, never 'love' or 'darling'; never to resort to the infantilizing collective pronoun – 'how are we doing today?' It seems a small thing but the language we use is subtly powerful in shaping our attitudes; to address someone with courtesy and formality acts as a corrective against objectification, diminution, even a kind of unconscious derision.)

To age is a process that doesn't just ruffle the vanity but agonizes the ego, because it brings 'the contradiction between inner and outer of a different order to anything we have previously faced'.

Montaigne described old age as a 'special favour' and 'privilege'. But – until he sent King Lear to rage upon the heath, to descend into madness and earn a new and revelatory kind of sanity – Shakespeare's old characters are almost invariably pompous, tedious or feeble, appearing as comic interludes, walk-on fools. Dickens usually puts his old characters in dark corners; they are the misers and mad people, spontaneously combusting out of pure rage, or they are the saccharine and the saintly from whom all desire and restlessness has leaked away. In films, the old are mostly notable for their absence, or are cameo parts and supporting characters. In fiction and in real life, the general rule of thumb is that the older people get, the more invisible they become; and when they do make themselves visible they are often regarded as a bit batty, if potentially endearing.

Becoming old is seen as a story of deficit and loss. The sense of decay provokes fear, disgust and a kind of recoil. 'Please, *please*, don't talk about old age so much, my dear old friend. You are giving me the creeps!' wrote Elizabeth Bishop to her friend and fellow poet Robert Lowell, adding, 'I wish Auden hadn't gone on about it so in his last years, and I hope you won't.' 'The creeps': something unseemly then, something weirdly shameful, on a different track entirely from inevitable decline.

In youth and health, 'it is all there to hand,' says Raymond Tallis to me: 'the size of the world, the available world, the community of the mind'. Youth gives us 'alacrity' and 'abundance'. It is about possibility; you are eligible for everything. When I was young I had the feeling that all that happened – however bruising; however sad – was part of the formation of myself. Rejection, divorce, failure, humiliation, all the setbacks and ambushes of life: I was under construction and they were materials. Now I've begun to feel that my ramshackle, cobbled-together house is pretty much built and I have to live in it, even if the tiles are loose, the windows rattle, and it's not the one I'd dreamed of. Living in the house I made, no one else to blame but me, one day not so far off I will be able to reach up 'and touch the ceiling' of my end.

'The story of ageing is the story of our parts,' writes Atul Gawande. 'Consider the teeth.' Yes, and consider the eyes, the hands, the knees, the hearing, the heart. Consider the skin – young, it is smooth and elastic; it fits us and holds us intact. But as we age, it sags and folds; pinch it and it no longer snaps back. We can no longer take our body for granted and repeatedly it lets us down. It *betrays* us. With the wear and tear of time, worn and eroded by life, we fail like complex systems fail, 'randomly and gradually'. Being old can seem to mean that 'something is not quite right'. Look at the advertisements in the magazines for older people: laxatives and aids for incontinence, stair lifts, walk-in baths, tonics and remedies for aches and pains . . . We want to avert it: buying face cream to reduce wrinkles, lured by the dentists' promise to restore the whiteness of a smile and turn back time, even going under the knife. We live in a culture where senility is scary in others and unacceptable in ourselves to a point where it is almost seen as an illness.

In his *New Yorker* piece about Silicon Valley's quest to live for ever, Tad Friend ironically evokes it as 'the creeping and then catastrophic dysfunction of everything, all at once. Our mitochondria splutter, our endocrine system sags, our DNA snaps, our sight, hearing and strength diminish, our brains fog, and we falter, seize and fail.'

It is for these reasons that Ezekiel Emanuel – distinguished oncologist, bio-ethicist, senior fellow at the Center for American Progress and author– is ready to die when he reaches the age of seventy-five; or at least, he no longer wants to struggle to keep alive, as he explains in his controversial article, published in the *Atlantic* in 2014. Under a beaming image of himself looking healthy and exuberant, he sets out his reasons for allowing nature to take its course. As a doctor, Emanuel has seen too many people holding on to life at all costs, until it is a ragged, tattered, excruciating thing. People are pumped full of drugs, plugged into machines, go under the knife, endure experimental treatment that makes their final months and years an agony of pain, hope and despair. Yet Emanuel is not simply saying that he doesn't want life at all costs, but that at a certain designated age – seventy-five – he will have lived to his fulfilled age and will no longer accept any kind of medical treatment. In his late fifties, fit and active and successful, he writes:

> I am sure of my position. Doubtless, death is a loss . . . but living too long is also a loss. It renders many of us, if not disabled, then faltering and declining, a state that may not be worse than death but is nonetheless deprived. It robs us of our creativity and ability to contribute to work, society, the world. It transforms how people experience us, relate to us, and, most important, remember us.

Emanuel turns to his seventy-seven-year-old father (two years beyond his own cut-off point) for an example: 'Once the prototype of a hyperactive Emanuel, suddenly his walking, his talking, his humor got slower. Today he can swim, read the newspaper, needle his kids on the phone, and still live with my mother in their own house. But everything seems sluggish . . . no one would say he is living a vibrant life.' (It should be said that Emanuel senior, whose life is being downgraded, explicitly says that he is happy, and his life sounds just fine to me.) Emanuel is also concerned that 'our living too long places real emotional weights on our progeny . . . Unless there has been terrible abuse, no child wants his or her parents to die. It is a huge loss at any age. It creates a tremendous, unfillable hole. But parents also cast a big shadow for most children.' He wants his own children to remember him as 'active, vigorous, engaged, animated, astute, enthusiastic, funny, warm, loving.

Not stooped and sluggish, forgetful and repetitive, constantly asking "What did she say?" We want to be remembered as independent, not experienced as burdens.' At seventy-five and beyond, he says, 'I will accept only palliative – not curative – treatments if I am suffering pain or other disability.'

This places enormous value on being active and vigorous, no value at all on being slow and full of years. When he talks of the diminution that occurs in old age, he is talking about power: not just material, worldly power but the power that Raymond Tallis evokes when he talks of the world 'being at hand'. He is strong in his own body (at the time he wrote the piece he had just climbed Kilimanjaro) and in his mind, at the peak of his career, obviously surrounded by family, friends, colleagues, operating on multiple levels. He is like one of those imaginary figures that have electricity crackling from their fingertips, at the centre of an intricate web of connections, the charged world pouring into them and rippling out of them, marvellously, vibrantly, powerfully alive and in charge.

I first read the piece shortly before my father died, when I was witnessing someone I loved living beyond his time. Then, I think I was most struck by its good sense. Three years later, I am unsettled by its vigorous certainty. What is missing is an account of vulnerability. To be human is to be dependent; this isn't a weakness but a necessary condition of being alive. We are born helpless and we die helpless, and in between is the continual flux of giving and receiving, of being at each other's mercy, of helping others and being helped in our turn. 'The body ages. The body is preparing to die. No theory of time offers a reprieve here. Death and time were always in alliance.'

Death and time: the unruly acceleration of old age over-turns the progress narrative. The concept of decline is the story of the body. The prejudice against old age is born out of a horror at decay. (When I was little and my grandmother came to visit I used to be properly terrified of seeing her naked. If she was in the bathroom, the door shut, I would feel squeamish at the thought of her in there, the folds of the sagging body.) But we should not think of old age as pathological, or a disease that can be cured. Decline is part of who we are; we are always impermanent, always growing towards our end, and old age is part of what gives life its necessary boundary and shape. The awareness of change and mortality, which can feel vertiginous and unendurable, is at the same time what gives us selfhood, and life meaning. It is the pattern of growth and decay that makes our existence bearable (though it can feel unbearable). Life has meaning precisely because it is a process. It begins and it ends – for everything that has a beginning has to have an ending. We can only have a sense of self if we know the self will age, and the self will die.

'Take care,' I would say when taking my leave of my dear friend Nick when he was old and frail. And he would glare at me: 'I certainly will not.'

If life is an adventure, old age perhaps demands the most courage and endurance.

'Take care,' I say to my mother.

She is in her mid-eighties and a widow after sixty-one years of marriage. She has always been a vivid personality, extrovert and captivating, but in the year after my father died she became distressingly muted. She seemed like a flame turned down very low, almost extinguished by grief and loneliness. Then, with an effort I now see was heroic, she took herself in hand, throwing herself back into life. Home had always meant my father: she was twenty when they met, and until his death had never lived alone. Bereavement has given her an existential restlessness. She went to live abroad in order to learn French, had singing lessons after a lifetime of being pronounced tone-deaf, and developed an unnerving habit of running down hills (blindly) in the middle of the road because she likes to feel the wind in her face and likes to feel free (and to astonish). She pays no attention to our cautions, which alarms and pleases us. She clambers up ladders. She travels to Angola to visit my sister. When I asked her recently, if I asked her to climb Everest with me, would she agree, she said, 'Yes!', her face lighting up as if I might be serious. She wants to learn to scuba dive. Her impulse for adventure is a form of self-preservation: it's her way of staying alive.

'You have to be tough to be old,' she says to me. Or perhaps: 'You have to be old to be tough.' Both, I think.

But really, strong or weak or wise or foolish, you just have to be old to be old. For the rest of us, it's a foreign country that we travel towards and will if we are lucky come to in our time.

3. The Brain, the Mind and the Self

'the marvel of consciousness – that sudden window swinging
open on a sunlit landscape amidst the night of non-being'

'Something is wrong,' my father said to me, before he could no
longer say anything. Sitting on the side of his bed and staring
down at his unlaced shoes: 'I don't know what's wrong. Something. What?'

What does one say to such a question? *Nothing is wrong?*
(Everything is.) There is such an urge to reassure: *You'll be all
right.* (You won't.)

Or this: *There is something wrong with your brain. You have a
complex brain disease. There is no cure.*

'Do you want to hold it?'

I nod. The room is bright and cool, full of stainless-steel
surfaces, large fridges and freezers that mildly hum, white
plastic tubs and Tupperware on shelves in which pieces of the
body float in liquid. It looks like a canteen, but without any
ovens.

I take the brain. It is heavier than I expected, softer: a gelat-
inous, pale mass. This soft, inert thing used to be the seat of
a self; it contains around 86 billion nerve cells, a dot the size
of a sugar grain containing about 10,000 and each one connecting to about 10,000 others, avidly consuming energy and
giving life and meaning, magnificently plastic and connective

and dynamic, never asleep even when we are, a miracle of perpetual motion with the body as its battery.

It's usually compared to a walnut, Shakespeare's 'nutshell'. It looks like a foetus, like two clenched fists. It looks like slimy coils of tripe, bloodless, folds within folds. It's impossible not to think of food. And when Steve Gentleman takes a long knife and cuts the brain in half (two observers at this point leave the room, rustling in their paper robes), it looks like a cross-section of cauliflower florets, but with a texture like spam or tofu.

With immense delicacy, Steve Gentleman carves the brain into thin slivers, laying them side by side along the surface.

Here is the left hemisphere; here the right. Here is the hippocampus, named after the seahorse for its curled shape, where long-term memories are stored, and also the memory of objects and people. These holes aren't really holes (there aren't holes that our memories fall through), but shrinkages so that the ventricles become larger. Here at the stem is the crucial medulla oblongata, which controls involuntary functions (breathing, controlling blood pressure). This is the cerebellum, responsible for balance and for voluntary tasks (like reading and writing). Here's the pons, the bridge between the upper and lower brain. This gluey blob that looks a bit like a white tadpole is the olfactory nerve. This is the amygdala, responsible for the memory of emotions, especially fear. Here is hunger; here is desire; here is speech; here is spatial awareness. Here is music, imagination, intuition, creativity, insight. Here is reasoning, logic, analytic thought. Here is damage. Look. The blade points. And here.

Here is loss.

Steve Gentleman (the name is accurate), Professor of Neuropathology in the Department of Medicine at Imperial College

London, is a detective of the brain. He looks for disease, shrinkage, hollows, hardening, white lesions in the limbic system, amyloid deposits. I ask him if he ever feels – I struggle for a right word, can't find it – *odd* about dissecting brains: odd because of what it tells us about identity, and because in the end all the urgent business of being human, all the despair, anxiety, appetite, terror, love and joy, resides in this piece of flesh.

He smiles and shakes his head. He has no faith – perhaps it would be hard to if day after day you slice brains, scalpel out morsels of executive function, episodic memory – but he is full of wonder at how infinitely complex, subtle and plastic the brain is, and how it is still mysterious to us. Because, after all, we are not just our brain: our brain is in a body, is part of it and in the community. There's no end to its possibilities.

Alzheimer's disease leads to nerve-cell death and tissue loss in the brain. Abnormalities include beta-amyloid plaques, tangles of the protein tau, loss of connection between the cells and inflammation. The cortex shrivels up and the ventricles grow larger. Over time the brain shrinks dramatically until every area is affected. Yet some brains, when dissected, show no sign of dementia even when the person has been diagnosed with the illness, while others are badly damaged even though the person seemed not to have shown signs of cognitive impairment. The link between observable deterioration in the brain and the way a person acts, feels and communicates in the world is not straightforward, and this is because the brain lives and works in a network of reciprocal connections. Looking at the brain cannot tell us all we need to know about the brain: it is so much more than itself – a brain in a body in a particular life. Part of Steve Gentleman's research is to compare the brain that he observes with the lifestyle of the man or woman to whom it belonged, to seek out patterns that will begin to explain why it is that some people are swiftly demolished by the illness when others are able to withstand its attacks for longer. Exercise, diet, geography, career, mood, the state of a relationship: all these things may make a difference to the way a person responds to what is happening in the intricately folded labyrinths of the brain.

The brain on its chopping board is inert, a lifeless beige thing, but neuro-images of the living brain display its fizzing connectivity, its marvel and mystery. Functional magnetic resonance imaging (fMRI) measures brain activity by detecting changes associated with blood flow. The images – still and moving – are like the Northern Lights, like coral reefs or trees in blossom, in kaleidoscopic flux. It may seem, looking at these iridescent patterns, that here's a brain in love, in fear, in envy and in a clutch of hope. But brain-scan images are not straightforward photographs of the brain in action; they are representations of the areas that are working at their hardest. It's a bit like looking at New York City from a helicopter and seeing how the crowds move through the streets: you learn a lot about the movement of people over time and in response to events, but you don't really know what it's like to be in New York. And the brain is not the mind.

Nevertheless, the image of a brain damaged by dementia is dismaying: dead grey patches amid the glorious colour.

'I do *not* like the term "dementia".'

I met Professor Martin Rossor in his room overlooking Queen Square in London, with windows from floor to ceiling. He is the National Institute for Health Research National Director for Dementia Research, Director of the Queen Square Dementia Biomedical Research Unit, Professor of Clinical Neurology and

Consultant Neurologist at the National Hospital for Neurology and Neurosurgery. He's tall and slim, with grey hair and a courteous manner. His cleverness is unintimidating; when he talked to me, he was pragmatic, precise and kind.

' "Dementia" is a catch-all phrase. It's powerful, but it's unhelpful for clinicians and scientists. It just means cognitive impairment that's so great that the person is badly affected.' There is not a 'uniform' breakdown of the brain but 'islands of breakdown'.

Dementia is a syndrome. It describes a set of symptoms of impairment in memory, communication and thinking caused when the brain is damaged by disease and is an umbrella term for a great range of progressive conditions that affect the brain. As Martin Rossor was at pains to emphasize, there are multiple forms of dementia and so there are multiple indicators of the disease. Alzheimer's is the dementia that people are most familiar with and accounts for over half of those affected by dementia. It is a neuro-degenerative disease that sweeps inexorably through the brain: the build-up of tangles and sticky clumps known as plaques used to be thought the cause of brain dysfunction, but scientists now think they may instead be like ash after a fire. Alzheimer's tends to develop gradually over time and is strongly associated with memory loss, poor concentration, confusion, the decline of everyday living skills. Other dementias – such as vascular dementia, which develops when arteries delivering blood to the brain become blocked, commonly after a stroke – frontotemporal dementia, or dementia with Lewy bodies, have different causes and different effects. Frontotemporal dementia, for instance, affects behaviour and personality, sometimes bringing about disinhibition, inappropriate social behaviour, anxiety, stress, even psychosis. And dementia can be a trigger for other mental-health conditions – such as depression – that can too easily be missed.

Even within a particular form of dementia, there are huge variations. Martin Rossor used the example of Alzheimer's: it commonly presents itself as loss of episodic memory and threatens the sense of selfhood that comes from a feeling of continuity between the you of ten or twenty years ago and the you of today. Yet there is a form of Alzheimer's in which memory is largely preserved but visual processing is damaged. Colours extend beyond their boundaries; things seem upside down; you can't locate objects; can't find the door. Often people feel that they are standing at an angle. Or they see a small puddle and think it's a hole. Or, standing at the top of an escalator, they stare down a gushing waterfall. Or reach out to grasp a handle that is in fact several metres away. 'I had a friend who had dementia who would grip on to things very tightly: it wasn't, as people assumed, resistive behaviour but because he thought he was falling.'

There are a bewildering number of cognitive impairments that come under the umbrella term of 'dementia', in part because there are so many kinds of memory, as Steve Gentleman demonstrated with the tip of his knife. (In one book, I read that, at the last count, there were 256.) Take the loss of semantic memory, Professor Rossor said: frontotemporal dementia is a 'horrible degenerative disease' in which a person loses the memory of the 'meaning of things'. Pick's disease, on the other hand, brings about the loss of verbal memory.

'Let's imagine you have a verbal semantic memory impairment. You would remember coming here, crossing the square. You'd remember I wore spectacles for reading. But if I asked you what spectacles were, you'd have no idea what I was talking about.' This incomprehension spreads until 'there is no comprehension of the human word or any output of language' – and with this pouring away of meaning, empathy will also go.

Other people may lose the memory for visual semantics. They 'understand the word "spectacles" but they have no idea what they are when they see them. They would know what a toothbrush was, but they might clean their teeth with the toothpaste tube. The world is breaking selectively around meanings.'

Symptoms can encompass great areas of loss, or be viciously precise: for instance, there's a dementia that can cause anosognosia, where people who are cortically blind nevertheless believe that they can see.

I asked Martin Rossor if he believes that a self is ever wholly lost to the disease, and he pondered. 'Perhaps when all empathy goes,' he replied eventually. 'Perhaps then.'

I asked him – as I will ask all those I speak to who witness the ravages of the disease – if he was scared of dementia himself. He hesitated and then answered that he was not and looked slightly surprised at the answer.

I asked what he makes of advance directives – the legal documents in which a person specifies what actions should be taken for their health if they can no longer make decisions for themselves because of illness or incapacity – for those who live with dementia. He nodded, frowned. 'How can I dictate to my future self?'

'Every death is terrible but we have to die. Your last years of life: how do you want to spend them? As the person you were or as a person who wouldn't recognize that self any longer? Who takes their child for their brother or sister – at their good moments? My life is the life of a thinking person. That is me. If that ends, my body should also end . . . That's why we made our living wills.'

In a tall, lovely old house in Utrecht, gable-roofed and full of flowers, every wood-panelled room lined with books, rich yellow light falling through the high windows, Gerard de Vries and Pauline Terreehorst talk to me about their decision to appoint each other in their living wills as the one who – if necessary – will confirm to the doctor that they want to die in dignity, should the conditions they have specified in their living wills manifest themselves. She was once a newspaper journalist and columnist and is now a successful director of an arthouse movie theatre; he is a distinguished philosopher, recently retired, who used to advise the Dutch government in The Hague. They are calm, dispassionate, carefully precise as they talk about their arrangements, which are already in place. Assisted dying for patients who are enduring unbearable suffering with no prospect of improvement has been legal in the Netherlands since 2002, provided the doctor complies with the 'due care' conditions set by the law. Among other things, he or she has to be sure that the patient's request for euthanasia is voluntary and well considered. Increasingly, it is acknowledged that not only physical but also mental suffering may be unbearable.

Of course, it's a controversial issue, regarded by many as the slippery slope that can end in the murder of the old – above all because of the issue of voluntariness. How can a person with dementia make an autonomous decision about ending their life?

'There is no un-clarity,' says Gerard firmly. 'In the later stages of dementia, the notion of a "voluntary, well-considered decision" is void. So, the wish to die with dignity should have been articulated well before those stages, in the limited time slot between being diagnosed with Alzheimer's and the stages in which one will have become mentally incapable.'

'I am sure, quite sure, that I want this,' adds Pauline. 'Our life was and is the life of thought. When that goes, well – it's no longer our life.'

As we talk through the evening, sitting first in their living room, then over a meal in their kitchen (fish baked individually in foil, like little gifts), they pass the conversation about their end-of-life between each other, following threads, correcting any imprecision. They both have a dread of incapacitated and impaired old age, and in part this is because of their very different personal experience of it. Gerard's father did not have dementia, but he had a serious stroke.

'He lay there, unable to speak, but he clearly signalled non-verbally he wanted to go. The doctor provided palliative care and let him die.'

His mother lived for many years more, her final ones in a home where she was well cared for, much visited, but her world was shrinking until, at some point, says Gerard, she must have thought, 'We're done here'. When, two weeks shy of her ninety-third birthday, she got pneumonia, she declared that she did not want to be treated.

'She wasn't depressed; she was clear in her mind. She said it to me and she said it to my brother and my sister: she was adamant that she had reached the end of her life and now was simply sitting, waiting to die. It was hard – but at no point did I try to make her change her mind. She was brave. And she died when she was still in control of her life.'

She said her goodbyes – she told Pauline to take good care of Gerard, her boy. And then she slipped away.

Both of Gerard's parents decided when they were ready to go. Neither of Pauline's parents did. When she talks about them she is tense with emotion. Time has not smoothed over the memories.

Pauline's father – with whom she had a complicated

relationship after he and her mother divorced, although when she was little she adored him and he her – was sixty-five when he started showing signs of the illness. He was forgetting small things but was able to cope for a while. Bit by bit, he slipped through the stages of dementia. He spent the last six or seven years in a nursing home – 'an awful one' – where he shared a room with another man.

'He had nothing left,' Pauline says. 'There were just a few photos around his bed. And he was –' She pauses. 'A plant. I would say that, yes. He lay in bed. He could do nothing. His wife visited him; we visited him. It was a Christian nursing home. In some places, he would have been allowed to die, but there, life was sacred. He was nursed to the bitter end.'

Pauline's mother is still alive; in fact, she is in a home just a few minutes' walk away from this house where we sit in the dusk, drinking wine. Her dementia started about ten years ago, although the symptoms were horribly muddled up with the difficulties in her marriage. Her third husband had suffered a stroke, which had changed his character. He could not cope with Pauline's mother's disease, her absent-mindedness; their final years together were filled with ugly minor quarrels, a sense of life tangling up and become disorderly. Pauline's mother used to be a member of the Union for Euthanasia and had always insisted she would like to die before dementia took its grip on her. But the window of opportunity for such decisions is very small: she missed her chance and is now in the deep darkness of the illness.

'It's like she's the living dead,' says Pauline. 'A long time ago, I lost her. I talk, and there's no reaction. Sometimes, when she laughs, or something in the tone of her voice – then I recognize the way we were twenty years ago. You fill in the gaps and the memories. Then she leaves again. You say goodbye all the time.'

'The thought,' says Gerard, 'of ending my life like Pauline's parents is quite appalling to me. We knew we were reaching the age when we had to face such questions.'

I am impressed, unsettled. The present self is making a decision about the future self – but what if the future self does not agree? What if, when they arrive at this conjectural time of diminution, wreckage and loss, they are content and have no wish to die?

They nod. 'It's a pre-binding of the self,' says Gerard. 'Just as countries have constitutions.'

'So if the future you,' I ask, 'says that you want to live after all – what then?'

'If Gerard is able to communicate his wish to live, no doctor will perform euthanasia. What we are talking about is the discussion we need to have in the limited time slot between diagnosis and the later stages of Alzheimer's,' Pauline replies calmly. 'Then I'll help him by reminding him of his past self. If we let that opportunity go, in the later stages of Alzheimer's only the option of refusing treatment will be available. Because Gerard has appointed me as his representative, I will point out to the doctor that in these circumstances that is what he – his former self – had wished.

'But,' I say. 'But *could* you?'

'I take as my example Odysseus and the Sirens,' Gerard says. 'His sailors bound him to the mast of the ship and he told them that however much he cried out, begging to be released, they should not do it.'

They look at me with kind expressions.

'We have to love each other a great deal to do this,' says Pauline, and I'm reminded of how a friend said to me recently that she would be unable to end the life of her mother, who has advanced dementia, because they had a difficult and damaging relationship and she does not love her enough to kill her.

So Pauline and Gerard have chosen to write a statement, each on the same day, stating their conditions, which are basically the same, and they have discussed their statements with their doctor, to whom they reconfirm their commitment every year. They have named each other as their first representatives and Pauline's daughter and Gerard's son as their second.

Gerard says that writing this down is lifting a burden from their children: 'It's not their decision; you are removing the burden of the very painful decisions that they would otherwise have to make.' The crucial thing, he says, is that he is deciding under certain conditions that he does not want to live. He is *asking* Pauline to grant him that wish; he is *asking* the doctor. 'It's a request.'

They are tranquil and stern, talking about the way they want to die, very sure that at a certain point a life is 'completed' and fulfilled: you cross a line, which is not the line that separates life from death, but the self from its own self-knowledge. 'Identity is not a kernel inside yourself; what we call our "identity" is the *outcome* of our actions, decisions, our personal and professional life, not their *source*. One's "self" is a network of social relationships, all one's attachments. The idea that identity is something *in* us, *inside* us, is part of a Christian heritage. We know as we get older the networks shrink. If they shrink beyond a certain point, your life no longer has meaning.'

On the opening page of *Admissions*, a wry and elegiac account of his life in medicine, the neurosurgeon Henry Marsh writes of the suicide pack he keeps at home, ready for when he is diagnosed with a disease such as dementia. He sees himself as a 'transient electrochemical dance, made of myriad bits of information', and his work has continually forced him to confront the changeability of personality because of damage in the brain. He wants to die before this happens to him.

Hugo Claus, one of Belgium's most renowned writers, best known for the novel *The Sorrow of Belgium* and his caustic portrayal of his country, was diagnosed with Alzheimer's disease in his late seventies. On 19 March 2008, in the Middelheim Hospital in Antwerp, he died by euthanasia, choosing the time and the place of his death. Friends said that he wanted to depart with dignity and pride. 'He left us as a great glowing star right on time, just before he would have collapsed into a stellar black hole.'

On 20 May 2014, Sandy Bem, a Cornell psychology professor in her sixties, took her life after careful preparation. She was a person whose identity was intimately entwined with her capacity to think and to write, and her diagnosis of Alzheimer's filled her with terror at the prospect of becoming 'hollowed out' by the illness, with no memory or sense of identity. She also hated her powerlessness in the face of the illness: 'She wanted to squeeze in as much intellectual and emotional joy as she could before she died, but she wanted to make sure she didn't wait too long. She needed to be engaged enough in her life to be able to end it.' It is extraordinarily difficult for one's body to die in tandem with the death of one's sense of self; she made a vow that she would take her own life before she lost this sense. She kept a journal that tracked her decline, and she talked to her ex-husband, who had remained her close friend, and to her children, telling them of her decision. 'What I want,' she typed in her journal in an emphatic boldface font, 'is to die on my own timetable and in my own non-violent way.'

She read books to find out gentle ways to die, she continually reaffirmed her decision to take her own life, she became a grandmother, which gave her great joy, she spent much time with her ex-husband, and she gradually declined, until it became clear that the suicide window was closing and, before long, she would no longer be able to make a decision about ending her life. And at this point she chose a month – May, when the world would be beautiful again, after the winter – and a date, Tuesday 20th. She wrote her death-day on the calendar that hung in her kitchen. She was deteriorating rapidly: a time came when she asked her sister who that woman was who'd just been with them. She was Sandy's daughter. Two days before the date she was to die, her family held a party for her, full of reminiscences about her life. ('Did I really do that?' she would say, pleased.) On Tuesday, 20 May, just as she had planned, she took her drugs of choice with a glass of wine, her ex-husband sat with her, and soon she fell into a sleep. The family were summoned and they watched her breathing and then they watched as the breathing stopped.

The psychiatrist Paul Wolfson did it alone. When he was diagnosed with a rare form of early-onset dementia that erodes the ability to think and speak he was sixty, happily married to his second wife, Lore Windemuth, with two small children. Over several months, he and his wife recorded their discussions about his illness, his slow and relentless decline, their radically altered future. He dreaded going into residential care but equally hated to think of himself still at home, his two young children seeing him 'pissing and shitting', and a carer there to 'contain' him. He foresaw the time – coming towards him swiftly – of not recognizing his children, not caring about them, not caring about his wife, 'only caring about myself . . . It's not brilliant, is it?' And so, aged sixty-one, he took his life. He did it with great thought. His wife took the children out for the day and when she returned he was dead. On the table beside him was a photo of his parents. He had left flowers for her and a Valium on her bedside table. So he departed from those he loved, in an act of generous love.

I have long believed that for many people, especially those living with dementia, life lasts longer than it should and becomes a cruel burden both for the subject and those who care for them. We should be better able to choose when to take our leave. Yet against the calm certainty and rationality of Gerard and Pauline, the decisiveness of Sandy Bem and Paul Wolfson, I have to set the tiny, dashing figure of Theresa Clarke, a woman with dementia who crackles with the desire to live life to the hilt and possesses a radical optimism that can seem like a kind of fury.

The first time I meet her is in Heathrow Airport. My train is held up and I am late to arrive. As I hurry to Arrivals, a miniature woman with silver hair races towards me, clattering a bag behind her, her eyes glittering, one hand lifted, on her face a look that in its intensity of excitement and fear is almost feverish. I hold up my hand in greeting and she spins to a halt, gives a full-throttle laugh, flings her arms around me. She has flown, unaccompanied, from Antrim to talk at a conference about dementia that is to take place the following day. I am small, but I tower over her. And I'm bowled over by her: her courage and determination, the way she wants to immerse herself in life, her refusal to give up on herself or be scared.

Theresa is the daughter of an Irish labourer, the eleventh of thirteen children, educated in the school of hard knocks. Though her father died when she was four, she remembers him vividly – running to meet him, 'and he would put me on his shoulders and away we'd go'. After his death, the family were very poor. Her mother – all these years later, Theresa still talks of her with a fierce protectiveness – worked in a munitions factory and as a cleaner. But Theresa remembers her childhood as 'full of fun'. If her mother had a spare 'roughness' (a coin), she would take them all to the seaside for the day or take a tram to the end of the Falls Road and have a sandwich. She remembers being interested in everything: she was a 'tomboy', a footballer. The boys would call at her house and say, 'Can Teasie come and play?' She tells me this and I can picture her as that child, wiry and quick, fierce with hunger for life.

She always wanted to be a nurse, and she always wanted to travel: 'A new country, a new job, new people: I've always been a seeker.' She has worked as a psychiatric nurse and a midwife (the 'most glorious job'), and she has lived in Cyprus, Australia, in Arctic Canada, in America. She loved to camp, to hike. She lived in an ashram in India for seven years. 'I wanted to be free. Twice I was engaged – people expected you to marry. But I'm so glad I held on to my freedom. A free bird.' She worked on social justice projects ('standing for myself, standing for others'), wrote poetry, was a bit of a hippy, a bit of a mystic. It seems to me that she's a woman who has always hurled herself at experience, chin up, plucky (as Helena says of Hermia in *A Midsummer Night's Dream*, 'though she be but little, she is fierce'). Her mother once told her that she had 'a heart like a lion'.

Ten years ago, Theresa Clarke's wandering ended. She came back to Northern Ireland and lived in the Glens for a few happy years with her beloved dog, moving to Antrim when she had heart trouble. In 2010, she was diagnosed with dementia. But she already knew. 'Oh yes!' she gleams. 'I knew *just* what it was. I knew I was forgetting things. I knew there was a wrongness in the way I was thinking. My dog knew as well. She would look at me when I made a mistake: she had different looks for different mistakes and I always understood what she meant. Well, well: you have to face up to whatever you find in yourself.'

She knows that she is beginning not to know and that the not-knowing is getting worse. She will stop mid-sentence and stare blankly, waiting for the strangeness to recede and saying, 'Where am I? It will come back, it will come back.' She has a phrase she uses quite a lot to cover the lacunae: 'something of that ilk'. Whenever I ring her, which I do fairly often, she greets me with a bark of surprised laughter and then more or less the same words: 'Nicci, where have you been? I thought you had disappeared off the face of the earth.'

She feels the illness *here* – she bangs on her head with the heel of her hand. 'The brain power is running out; things disappear. It's a muddle and I get so tired.' But *here* – and she raps at her chest, as if the door to her heart can open wide – she remains herself. 'I am me, here, now.'

When I visit her in Antrim I see on her noticeboard, among multiple reminders and exhortations, the message: 'You are not this body; you are not this mind.' (The others include: 'Switch off electrical appliances!' 'You're doing well, keep it up.' 'Take your meds.' 'Nicci is coming on Friday.') She does 'walking meditations', pacing her miniature living room and garden, saying to herself, 'I am calm, I am smiling. The present moment is a wonderful moment.' Her insistence both impresses me and makes me uneasy: I wonder if she is hanging on to the notion of life's bounty by her fingertips, and if what she calls joy is actually her way of coping with despair. I don't know.

At the conference, Theresa talked eloquently about how people with dementia are too often treated as if they no longer had a stake in their own lives. 'We can still contribute to society, our family and the world beyond,' she declared in her quick-fire voice – she talks as if rushing to get a sentence out before she loses its thread. 'But for this to happen, we need to be part of the conversation about dementia: not just spoken about, like an object, but talked with and to.' Later in the day, she took part in a round-table discussion with several of the leading spokespeople in the field and was smiling, proud, diminutive, indomitable, sure of her place at the table.

Gerard and Pauline believe that the self exists in a rich and intricate network of connections and relationships; to be alive is to have a narrative of your life, with a past to reach back into and draw upon, and a future to anticipate and project on to. For them, identity involves self-consciousness, memory, language, rationality, all things that are gradually dismantled in dementia. But for Theresa, the self is 'not just my brain, not just my memories, much more than my experiences. I'm here, in the moment, alive and whole.' She is aware that her world is shrinking and the horizons are closing in: once, she travelled the globe, followed her questing spirit, went to the source of the Ganges. Once, she read books and wrote poetry. Today, her world is her little bungalow; her past dissolves behind her, everything she does during the day forgotten; her future is unknowable; the structures of her life have fallen away. 'But I'm still resonating,' she says. 'In the present. Now.'

Sean and I often talk about what we would do if we got dementia. After seeing what happened to my father, it's no longer an abstract question but an urgent, practical one. Would we want to choose our time of death? For a long time we have both supported someone's right to die if they have a terminal illness – and dementia is a terminal illness, after all; there comes a time when a person is no longer living with it but dying with it, becoming dead. The problem of course is that it is always too early – before you are ready to leave life but while you still have the capacity to make the decision – or too late; the departure gates have closed. And how do we make a decision for the unknown self we will become?

I'm struck that while both of us would want to accompany and care for the other – or we think that we would, which is something very different – we would not want to be looked after by the other, at the mercy of their kindness and the object of their pity and disgust. I'm also struck by how we talk about these possible selves who exist in the conditional future as dreaded *strangers*. The self of our childhood may feel starkly different from the self of our teenage years, and that self seems barely connected, save by memory and the story memory makes for us, to the self we become. Yet it feels continuous. For Raymond Tallis, 'It both is and it isn't. For instance, I still feel responsible for a mistake I made as a junior doctor in 1970. To be exact, 8 March 1970. I do believe it was the same person. There's a continuation of the body; there's a psychological continuation.'

We are attached to our past selves because we have been them and they are still lodged within us. All our infinite, shifting versions are contained by the present self – moment after moment, *now* and *now* and *now*, unquantifiably small fragments of experience piled up in the complex formation of the self. The child I was, the awkward teenager I was, the young mother ambushed by love, the woman in her thirties, her forties, have gone and the river of time runs on, and yet they are part of what made me. They are inside me, continually perplexed at my age and my wrinkles and my many follies and mistakes. We can't escape each other.

But the future self is a dizzying number of continually changing possibilities. To talk of a *me* in the future is just bewildering.

Not long ago, I uploaded a photo of myself on to an age-progressing app, which operates on the same principles used by forensic scientists to work out what missing children would look like today. A woman appeared on the screen: a small, wicked onion face, features barely distinguishable in a scrunch of wrinkle, mouth puckered in what might be the remnant of a smile but looks more like malice. Nope. That's not me. I refuse to become that mean old woman. I'll be someone different.

What is it to be a self, and where does the self end? Does it end with death or, in some cases – where a mind is picked apart by dementia – can it end before that?

The influential utilitarian philosopher Peter Singer has a list of indicators for 'personhood': 'self-awareness, self-control, a sense of the future, a sense of the past, the capacity to relate to others, concern for others, communication and curiosity'. This is a brutal catalogue that dismisses many people who do not possess such 'personhood'. In a society that places high value on reason, agency, memory, instrumental value, people with dementia count less or don't count at all – which in turn can mean that they are no longer treated with love, respect or dignity. If we lose the *sense* of our self – our self-consciousness, that which gives us our identity – do we also lose our self? Our value? Our reason to be alive?

'Neither *cogito* (I think) nor *ergo* (therefore) but *sum*: I am,' writes one passionate champion of the rights and the value of people with dementia, who believes that those with dementia have, individually and collectively, been deprived of their human dignity and respect because of our culture's increasing emphasis on autonomy, rationality and self-possession. This excludes 'the socially outcast, the unwanted, the marginalized and the oppressed'. People living with dementia become, over time and implacable decline, defenceless, powerless, easily victimized. At the end of their long life, at the time of their greatest need, they cannot speak for themselves. Our moral commitment should be to the vulnerable: fellow human beings on this little planet of ours.

When is it time to say goodbye and leave the party? Is there ever a point at which we cease to be ourselves and become 'a little piece of hell'?

During his last months, the disease attacked my father relentlessly on all sides. He had no way left to defend himself. I used to say that he had lost everything – but that's too simple. In some mysterious way, he did not lose his self. Somewhere inside John Gerrard there was always a John Gerrard. When people (me) reach after metaphors to describe what happens to a person with dementia, nothing quite fits. My father wasn't like a boat slipping its anchor and drifting out to sea – or not only. He wasn't like a landscape, ruined and the wind ripping through it; a city, bombed; a house, demolished; a deck of cards, shuffled; a glass, dropped; a manuscript torn into shreds.

Something is wrong. I don't know what's wrong. Something. What?

A complex brain disease, for which there is no cure . . .

He was like a man, an infinitely helpless and bewildered man, at the mercy of the world.

4. Memory and Forgetting

'All this goes on inside me, in the vast cloisters of my memory.
In it are the sky, the earth and the sea, ready at my summons . . .
In it I meet myself as well.'

My father might have been absent-minded, but he was very
good at remembering things: the speed of light, the dates of
battles, the periodic table, the Latin names of plants and the
English ones of wildflowers, the bones in the body, mathemat-
ical equations and chemical formulae, whole chunks of poems,
the colours of flags, capital cities . . . Then he began to forget
and the painstaking acquisition built up over a lifetime gradually fell away.

When did my father's dementia begin? We don't know. We'll
never be able to put a finger on the danger spot: *there*. Like fog
that creeps up stealthily, imperceptibly, until the foghorn
booms and suddenly there are dark shapes looming at you out
of shrouded darkness – you think you'll notice, but often you
don't. Then you can't.

I wonder when it began for my father, that unobtrusive slide
of memory, the wind going out of his sails. I'm sure my mother
sensed it before the rest of us. But what about him? When
did he hear the boom of the foghorn? Was he very scared? Was
he sad?

'Life without memory is no life at all.' Without memory,
things don't fit together; the narrative of one's life crumbles,

the walls of one's self tumble down. Without memory, you are adrift in a helpless present tense, and 'the world glides through you without leaving a trace'. How can we love without memory, have relationships, empathize or plan or imagine or anticipate, keep track of oneself, stand on firm ground? Memory as thought before thought and knowledge before knowledge; memory as a way of editing our own life; memory as a way of joining all our different selves together into a coherent whole; not a tool for thinking but an act of thinking; memory as a lie, a creation, a different kind of truth. Collective. Deeply personal. At war with death.

The terror of losing memories is the terror of losing the active self: that which holds us precariously together into the shape we have built up over our lives. To have and to make memories enables us to be the (often inaccurate, self-deceiving or misinformed) narrator of our own lives. Memories connect us to our past and launch us into our future; they link us to other people and bridge the labyrinths of the inner self to the abundance of the outer world. But memory's vast cloisters can crumble and fall into darkness; are the memories still in there, like restless ghosts, or have they been obliterated? Where, as Sally Magnusson asks in the title of her groundbreaking book about her mother's dementia, do memories go? And what are memories anyway?

In the summer of 2017, my mother and I revisited the house where our family lived for the first nineteen years of my life. It was something I had wanted to do for a long time. I drive past it every time I go to see my mother, and catching a glimpse through the trees my heart skips a beat: that was my past; there, half hidden, was where I used to be young. My siblings and I all grew up in the house; it was the architecture of our childhood, where we became the people we are. I had vivid memories of the place – too vivid, too sunlit, glowing with colour and replete with feelings; not just a home but a locus of selfhood and a place of innocence.

My mother and I went up the drive together and rang on the bell. They let us in.

Forty years had passed since we were here, and the house had changed a great deal. Walls had been knocked through and other walls built; rooms rearranged and joined together; trees chopped down and others grown tall. And inevitably, our memories had hardened into shapes that perhaps had more to do with how we wanted to remember those times than with reality. The two of us walked inside, stared about us, waited for something to happen.

Then, all of a sudden, at a twist in the stairs, the past gushed back so powerfully and purely that it didn't feel like memory. It felt like being there, being young again, and I was almost sick with longing and distress. And then again, those black and red tiles by the front door; that larder built into the sandstone; that cornfield by the side of the house that I used to run down with my siblings, and I was there once more, trying to keep up, bare, scratched legs and eyes full of the sky, and I could almost see our dog, Candy she was called, a golden retriever with sorrowful eyes. Now the house was full of ghosts. My mother stood by the window of the bedroom that used to be hers and my father's and she looked out at the garden, tears streaming from her nearly blind eyes, down her old and captivating face. Some memory is muscle-memory; much is voluntary – we search around for the memory, like opening drawers in the mind, make an effort to recall it. But here, memory was involuntary and engulfing, and felt more like a return to the past than a recollection of it. We were in the 'permastore' of long-term memory storage, where the past becomes ever more vivid. These flash-memories, which like lightning in the sky can suddenly illuminate a hidden landscape, strike everyone: they are a gift, an injury, seemingly random, triggered by the smell of sweet peas, a bar of music, the way light falls through the trees. Back come our former selves, unbearably familiar and yet almost strangers. Where have they been hiding all this time?

Sometimes I remember my father because I think about him; I make a hard effort to see his face or recall his words, summoning him back from the dead. Sometimes out of the blue he returns to me: when I see the birds come to our bird table (for he would always gather crumbs from a meal and put them out for the long-tailed tits and the finches). When I notice the wildflowers (he knew all their names and tried to teach me, though I retain only a few of them). When water boatmen skim across the surface of some pond or ditch. When I'm by a rock pool and it's almost as if he is suddenly beside me, peering into the crannies like a dreamy boy. Or looking at star-spangled skies and not knowing the names of constellations (but he would have). Or walking along overgrown footpaths and I remember how he would take his time tying back wayward brambles for walkers who might come after us. Moths knocking against the window with their powdery wings (he would catch them in his hands, carefully). Bees (he built habitats for them, to encourage them into the garden). Bonfires. A certain gesture. A figure in the distance (who isn't him). The sound of a chuckle. And there he is, unlooked for, alive again.

My father, in his years of forgetting, would gather stories about him in an act of self-protection. He had revisited them so often they were safe places for him. He didn't get lost in them: he knew his way around and was agile and sure. His path was worn smooth by repeated use, and nothing tripped him up or ambushed him, no shadows in the corners or craters to fall into. He had memories he could enter through any portal, wander around, touching familiar things, seeing them again, smelling pine trees and mushrooms and bonfire, fresh paint and the sea, hearing voices of old friends. His face would ease and look younger. He remembered being evacuated during the war and tramping the countryside; Finland and the saunas he took there; Egypt, where he was sent on his National Service; his university days. He remembered being carefree and youthful, just starting out – and the photographs of him when he was young show someone slim and buoyant, a zest about him. But bit by bit through those dementia years the gates of memory started to close; he would falter and stumble in the telling. There were fewer and fewer places he could enter, until finally, there was nowhere left to return to where the ground did not shift and ooze under his feet. No safe place.

We picture the memory as a place in which things are conserved and stored: a library, an archive, a chest, a wax tablet on which impressions are made and then rubbed away, a filing cabinet, a computer . . . Things are 'burnt' or 'imprinted' on to our memory. Trying to remember something feels like rummaging around in the attic of our mind, in dusty corners, in search of that elusive object: where have we put it? 'If only this could be your memory. A spacious room. Light falls through big windows. Everything is clean and orderly. Your memories stand in rows along the walls, meticulously updated.'

But memory is an 'an activity, not a vault . . . a process not a place': stored in different parts of the brain, memories are synchronized and work together 'like an orchestra'. Virginia

Woolf compares memory to a 'seamstress, and a capricious one at that', running her needle 'in and out, up and down, hither and thither', so that a whole ragbag of experiences is delicately, intricately joined together. And memories are no older than the last time they are thought of; 'there are no "read only" files'. To remember something is to create something new: it happens in the present tense, so that in the act of memory old selves are created afresh – the rough draft of a life that is being continually revised. Subjectivity is built into the very nature of memory. Memories are fallible, frail and representational – and at the same time, imaginative, flexible, creative and re-creative. They are the stories we tell others and tell ourselves, and they are the way we can recognize a self that persists over time.

Memory is always dominated by forgetting. If memory is the library or the cabinet, forgetting is the sieve, the thing with gaps – it's 'the minus sign' and 'exists within remembering like yeast in dough'. We have to forget or we will go almost mad with the overload, as is demonstrated by the sixty or so people identified thus far who possess the highly superior autobiographical memory known as HSAM. They can remember most of the days of their life as clearly as most of us remember the recent past. They can give the day and date thirty years ago, say, on which they did a particular exam, or tell you what the weather was like, what they and all their friends were wearing; they can remember a smell, a feeling, a mood . . . One middle-aged HSAM woman recalls a remark her mother made to her when she was a small child, and the memory brings back the flare of resentment that she felt all those years ago.

Memory needs its 'garbage heap'. Recent research has shown a connection between disturbed sleep and cognitive impairment. We have a nocturnal cleaning system (the glymphatic) that removes proteins called amyloid-beta, which accumulate into the plaques that contribute to Alzheimer's and dementia. During sleep, cerebrospinal fluid flows through the spaces between neurons, flushing proteins and other neural waste into the circulatory system and away. This is one reason why chronic insomnia is a risk factor for dementia. Another is that, in deep sleep, with its large, slow brain waves, fragile new memory traces are consolidated into more permanent forms of long-term storage. The memories initially encoded in the hippocampus are moved to other areas of the brain, clearing the slate, as it were.

The body is unimaginably complicated and clever. It 'knows' that the weight of remembering, the hoard of recollections, is an impossible burden. It knows we need to remember but we also need to forget. Sometimes when memory floods back pure and raw, as it did when my mother and I went to visit our old house, it can feel like a curse. Intense memory hurts; we need to recover from its injury. It does not feel like recollection – a dispassionate and voluntary pondering on past events – but more like an ambush from within, grabbing us, dragging us back to the past that we thought had vanished, or we thought we had escaped. Memory is also trauma; to forget the past is to lose our memory of loss. If love is intimately bound up with remembering, so too is grief. Love and grief and loss can over-whelm us.

My mother used to tell a story from her childhood: it was one among her collections of anecdotes, shaped and polished and taken out at family gatherings. In 1941, during the war, she was evacuated from Palestine with her mother and brother. She would have been nine. The ship they were on, the *Georgic*, was bombed in the Gulf of Suez and they were put in a life-boat, while behind them the ship slowly went down. My mother would tell us about the strong young sailor who picked her up and swung her over the side into the boat. And how when they were back on the safety of land a cry went up that someone's handbag had been found. The group of people, who had been leaving Palestine with all their worldly possessions on board, went eagerly to see whose it was – and of course, it was my mother's toy bag, containing no treasures.

That was the little story. I never really thought about what lay around its neat, domestic edges. Then a few years ago, out of the blue, she started to talk about another memory: the bombing had created a massive oil spillage on the surface of the sea. The water was on fire, and in the water – burning, drowning – were people crying out for rescue. Some of them she knew; they had been her neighbours and friends and now she saw their faces in the flames. But the lifeboats were already too full and so they rowed through the figures in the water. Her memory, her little story, was a screen against this terrifying episode; the bag had been a flimsy shield against the horror, but it had served her for a remarkably long time, until in age it would no longer do. We all have the stories that we polish and pass around, and we all have screen memories. But they can be fragile defences against the floods: my mother's story has ceased to protect her from what happened nearly eighty years ago. Now she remembers what she tried to forget and she dreams of people reaching out to her from the flaming water.

Remembering gives us our sense of self, our narrative, our identity. Forgetting keeps us sane. In dementia, this subtle negotiation between what we keep and what we let go of can break down. The distant past floods back, unmediated, with a freshness that can be joyful or tormenting, while the recent past fractures and disappears. Yesterday is swallowed up by darkness, but sixty years ago remains vivid. My father was lucky; he most often remembered saunas in Finland, carefree days at university. That old woman I saw in the hospital bed who was shouting out: 'No, no, please don't. Teacher, don't. It's down there' – she wasn't so lucky.

To lose one's power of remembering is not like losing a tool that is broken: you can look at the tool and see it is damaged, but here you *are* the tool; you *are* the process: forgetting wipes away the traces of itself. You don't notice the fog descending, though perhaps there is the warning boom in the gathering night. Things are gone without being missed; forgetting takes place unnoticed and you don't see that you aren't seeing. There is a special kind of terror in this silent obliteration that ploughs through the self like a furrow.

I read on a government website that you should seek advice and help if you: struggle to remember recent events, forget the names of friends and everyday objects, lose the thread of what you're saying, cannot recall things you have seen or heard, have problems thinking or reasoning, sometimes feel anxious, depressed or angry, get lost on familiar journey, often feel confused . . .

When I have no memory whatsoever of a film I saw the week before; when I find yoghurt on the bookshelf and crisps in the fridge; when I make the whole family look for my watch that I remember dropping on the floor somewhere in the house and then discover a few hours later is actually on my wrist, obscured by a long sleeve; when I order the same shirt online three times; when I carefully pour ground coffee into the little dishwasher capsule for soap; when I go upstairs for something but then have no idea what; when I point at the Thermos flask and call it a Tupperware; when I can't find my way home though I know I know the way; when I open the door and for one terrifying moment don't recognize the familiar face; when I look in the mirror and see my shirt is inside out and I only have one earring in; when I lose my supermarket trolley; when I can't remember where I parked; when my dreams leak into my day so I can't tell them apart; when I see people exchanging glances as I speak and realize that I'm repeating myself; when I have that sudden flushing awareness that I've somehow lost my grip on what's going on around me, the wind going out of my sails.

When does forgetfulness that is natural and part of getting older become something more sinister? How do we know when to be worried? When does the foghorn boom?

'Ah yes, worried-wellness,' says Sube Barnerjee wryly when I talk to him about how my middle-age forgetfulness always triggers the terror of dementia. He is an old-age psychiatrist and Professor of Dementia and Associate Dean at Brighton and Sussex Medical School who has served as the UK Department of Health's senior professional advisor on dementia. His research focuses on quality of life in dementia, and he is energetic, articulate, optimistic. 'Worried-wellness as in when I call my kid Sandy, which is actually the name of my dog. A life can be poisoned by the fear.'

Dr Claudia Wald is consultant psychiatrist at the Kensington & Chelsea and Westminster Memory Service, which provides dementia assessment and diagnosis and ongoing support for people with memory difficulties. Memory clinics like this are based on models from the US and were set up in the early eighties in every region of the country. She sits in her pleasant room, sunlight falling through the window. She is tall and open-faced, and her voice is reassuring; she feels a kind place to be.

'People of your age,' she says, 'start to fear their fading memories. With age comes effortful thinking and remembering': much forgetfulness is age-related and non-problematic. We all forget as we get older, and this is normal, natural, part of the ageing process. Dementia is not natural, it is a disease. Nevertheless, there is a grey area, a place of uncertainty and trepidation, when forgetfulness deepens – when, as so many people with dementia say, something seems 'not quite right'.

In her diagnostic work, Claudia Wald is looking for changes in behaviour. Almost always, the initial assessment is done in the person's home, where the atmosphere is more relaxed, less contrived, and where much can be learned from context (the state of the house, of the fridge). She takes a detailed clinical history and uses scans only where there is diagnostic uncertainty: 'I am trying to find out who the person was; I am looking for change.' She must assess what part of the memory is affected: long-term memory? Language? (The language centre is next to the memory centre.) 'The bank of words seeping away,' she says – then adds: 'This happens to us anyway.' Recalling names? Faces? In her diagnostic criteria, at least two domains must be affected (language and memory, say; or memory and behaviour; or memory and sense of direction), before she gives a formal name to the symptoms she finds.

Between the inevitable process of ageing and the clear diagnosis of dementia lies the swampy territory of mild cognitive impairment (MCI), an interim stage which some see as a pathologizing of natural forgetfulness and others as a helpful indication of future problems. For there is no scientific boundary between disease and normality; lines may be drawn, but their exact location is a matter of evaluative judgement. 'It's a grey area,' says Claudia Wald. 'And at what point in that grey area is treatment appropriate? What is "normal" as we get older?'

Often she will find that circumstances have changed, so that props are stripped away: the death of a spouse who had been compensating for failing cognitive function, going into hospital, breaking a leg, moving house. 'These things can expose difficulties that had been hidden.' Depression, she says, 'can be a precursor and a risk factor', and it can be very difficult to treat. 'Old age brings with it profound losses: the loss of a spouse, of family, of friends, of work, of health. There is huge loneliness and fear of death.'

All this means that the diagnosis is often not straightforward, and often it is the relative or carer who notices the change – because how can the *I* know that the *I* is slipping?

William Utermohlen, that thin and sad-faced man who became one of the great chroniclers of dementia's self-loss, did not know, or if he did he withdrew from the knowledge. He was living with his wife, Patricia, in their London flat overlooking the canal, a book-lined, painting-hung space where they both worked, he in the attic studio with a skylight. I sit in that flat now with Patricia, who is soon to be ninety, although she still teaches an art class and is eloquent and vital and pin-sharp. Her husband's paintings are on every wall; his face and hers stare down at me; the table at which they sit is the table at which I sit now.

She talks about her husband with tenderness and honesty: how he courted her (she had been married before, to a man she had been head-over-heels in love with, so was resistant at first); how they never had children and in some ways she was his mother-figure; how he never achieved the recognition he wanted. A figurative painter in a period when conceptual painting was dominant, he had some success in the early sixties but was then, in an exhibition of 1969, demolished by critics. He was 'destroyed', Patricia says, and perhaps he never quite recovered from the trauma, although the French art historian who represents Utermohlen believes that he started getting his energy back in the late eighties.

In the early nineties, several years before the official diagnosis, he became increasingly anxious. 'He was always an anxious man,' his wife tells me. 'But he became more and more so – and more withdrawn.' It was at this time that he began his 'Conversation Pieces', a series of paintings which French psychoanalyst Patrice Polini thinks were born out of a need to 'define his existential references and capture his familiar surroundings', and show a 'sense of urgency in the face of a gradually fading memory and disorientation'. Their titles – *Maida Vale, Snow, Bed, Night, W9* – fix the images in time and in space. These paintings are in many ways a celebration of the life that he and his wife shared: he returns over and over again to their large living room, flooded with light; through one window a view of the garden and another the canal, houseboats and the great city stretching out beyond. At the centre is always their table, at which Patricia sits, alone or with friends. Figures lean into each other, smoke cigarettes, drink wine, talk. There are cats (there are still cats); a rubber plant (and there is one still), coffee cups and wine bottles and ashtrays. The same decorated jugs stand on shelves. There are books everywhere. A sense of companionship fills the paintings – intimate talk is what these 'Conversation Pieces' evoke – and Pat is unequivocally at the centre. But it is possible to see the illness lurking, not just because some of the perspectives are starting to tip and solid objects are precarious, but because of the sense of the artist's loneliness. When he puts himself into his paintings, he is on the edge, a solitary and watchful figure; there's a painful sense of exclusion. He is painting himself out of the circle of warmth and vitality. In *Bed*, he shows Patricia sitting up, reading, cats winding their way about her; she's the painting's focus and it is on her that light falls, the vital centre. The artist lies next to her, on the far edge of the bed, the covers pulled over him so that only his small head is visible and there's no suggestion of a body attached to it. Is he dreaming? Is he awake? It's a profoundly troubling image. At the time it was painted, the disease was progressing in an 'underhand' way; he may have had a sense of it but he had no name for it. Just a sense of dread.

Patricia tells me of the watershed time he went to Paris, a city he knew very well, and got hopelessly lost. 'It shocked him deeply.' And shortly after that came another, much more ominous sign: he had been commissioned to do a family portrait for friends, grouped around their own table. 'For a whole year he sat in front of the canvas and he did nothing. Nothing. And then we knew.' He had always drawn, wherever he was. That was how he communicated. But now he had stopped dead. Pat thinks that he had some sense of what was happening to him before she did, but he did not say, could not say. He was still young. How could he have dementia?

Rebecca Myer's mother both knew and did not know. Rebecca is a nurse who works in the community, often with people with dementia. When she tells me her story, her manner is thoughtful and candid. She has a way of pausing after a question, thinking carefully before answering. Her thoughts take her back to a dark time, for the story of her mother's dementia is also the story of a close family struggling to manage chaos and disintegration. Her mother was an 'immensely gracious woman, thoughtful and kind'. She met Rebecca's father when they were both young, at an ice rink: 'she thought he was a show-off, twirling round and coming to a stop in front of her. Dad used to say that he wore her down.' They married when they were both twenty-one and were parents by the time they were twenty-two. 'They were *very* close,' she says. 'They'd hold hands in the back row of the cinema. I've a photo of them and they are just looking at each other and it says it all. The degree of loss,' she says, 'is relative to the degree of love.'

When Rebecca talks about the terrible years that tore her life in two, her face is bright with love and sorrow. Her mother was clever, and had been a grammar-school girl, but her parents had no expectations for her when she was growing up and she lacked confidence. She had part-time jobs and did voluntary work for a charity. She liked books, poetry, puzzles. She always read stories to her children and played games with them: Rebecca starts to tell me about a game of cat-and-mouse she and her mother used to play when as a tiny child she would help her mother make the beds – and then she stops and smiles. 'Strange what one remembers,' she says softly. 'So strange.'

'But what I really remember was that she was always there. When I came out of school, she'd be there; or later, when I came home from school on my own, she'd be there. When we watched TV, I'd sit by her and put my head on her shoulder. I'd tell her everything and she would listen to me for hour after hour. When I left home to train to be a nurse in London, I was very homesick. I missed them. I still miss them.'

Rebecca's mother was in her fifties when her family started to notice that something wasn't right. She had always been 'a worrier' but now she became more so, and was struggling. 'Now, in hindsight, I see there were signs,' says Rebecca. Her mother could no longer work out money. She couldn't measure out the formula for the baby milk for Rebecca's baby daughter. It was Rebecca's sister-in-law who eventually said:

'Your mum's not right; something's wrong.' But Rebecca's father was hiding it from everyone, and from himself: 'He just couldn't deal with the distress. Mum would say to him that she thought something was wrong, and he would tell her no, everything was fine, she wasn't to worry. His desire to protect us was incredibly strong.' And so he wouldn't confront what was happening in the heart of the family, and he wouldn't let her confront it either.

Tommy Dunne did not know. I visit him and his wife, Joyce, in Liverpool, where they live in a small, neat bungalow with flowers outside the front door and everything in its proper place – this is where they moved after he knew that he was ill, leaving their 'dream home'. He and Joyce sit together on a sofa, facing me as we talk, telling their story between them. They met each other when they were both sixteen, at a skating rink, like Rebecca's parents – though they weren't skating but going to an Edwin Starr concert. Tommy and his friend were sitting at the bar drinking (illegally). Joyce didn't fancy him at first; it was when she saw how kind he was to her baby sister that she started to take notice. They are both one of eight siblings and so they have a clan-like family in Liverpool. After they married, Joyce did odd jobs and Tommy worked on the railways, at first as a driver and then in management. Their son was born when they were just eighteen, their daughter several years later. They had, says Joyce, 'a good life. Everything was going the way we wanted.'

Tommy has a round face and is a man of smiles; he smiles as he talks now, but the years leading up to his diagnosis were hellish ones. His first symptoms were not of memory loss but of his world shrinking, and he takes out his iPad to pull up a diagram showing a series of concentric circles, each differently coloured ring representing aspects of an individual's world, from the bull's eye of *me*, to *family, friends, work, community, city* . . . 'The outer rings begin to fall away,' he says. He swipes left, left again. Circle after circle disappears.

Joyce joins in: 'I had noticed years before, perhaps as many as ten years before, that something was wrong. Tommy's job was quite stressful; he became absent-minded; got very quiet – he didn't speak as much as he used to. But I put it down to stress. You dismiss things and think, "Just get on with life." We didn't talk about it, but gradually I started to wonder if he had Alzheimer's. It wasn't just his memory. For example, we had this glass cabinet for appointment cards and things, and he couldn't see them. He couldn't find his coat when it was right in front of him.'

And then, 'One bad day at work' – Tommy goes on, smiling – 'I could feel it happening and I could see it. It was like one of those old films unravelling.' He makes a violent gesture with his hands. He stops talking.

'He shut down,' finishes Joyce for him. 'Completely shut down. I came home and he was lying in bed, shaking and shivering. I took him to the doctor and he was signed off for two weeks.'

Two weeks passed. Tommy went to see the work doctor who said, in front of him, 'This man will never work again.' He went to see the work psychologist, who thought he was having a nervous breakdown. Nothing changed. Tommy lay in his bed in a state of terror. Six months later, a psychiatrist diagnosed him as bipolar and he was put on lithium, gradually increasing the dose. 'I knew he wasn't bipolar,' says Joyce. 'He'd always been quick-tempered, but it wasn't that. I knew.'

Three times a day, he was visited by health professionals because he was believed to be a suicide risk. For a year, he lived with a sense of oppressive foreboding: 'A dread. I could feel it coming. Twenty-four hours a day. I thought I was going to explode, like a spring compressed and compressed and compressed inside me.' When Joyce left the house he would unplug the phone. If someone knocked at the door, he would go to bed and pull the covers over his head and wait for whoever was outside to go away. 'Time slowed right down. I was never going to get out of it, like a snowball rolling down a hill, worse and worse and worse.'

But he didn't know he had dementia.

Pauline's mother in the Netherlands did not know 'until that test drawing of the clock ... She was constantly laughing, fearfully, at the silly mistakes that she made.'

And my father? It's like mortality: until there's a test, a diagnosis, a name, knowing isn't *knowing*.

'You are no different the day after diagnosis,' says Sube Banerjee. 'Except that you recognize what you are facing.'

I nod. That's quite a large *except*.

'A diagnosis,' says Claudia Wald, 'is just the start of learning how to live well with this condition. There can be a paradoxical comfort from knowing there's a name and a reason for this changed sense of self, but some people do not want to know.'

I notice a subtle change in her manner. She picks up her pen: 'Are you ready?'

My racing heart, my sweating palms. It's like being back at school and doing an exam – except I am the exam that I don't want to fail.

'Remember these words,' she instructs. ' "Apple", "penny", "table". I will ask you for them later.'

I nod. *Apple, penny, table. Apple, penny, table.*

'I am going to give you an address which I want you to remember. David Barnes, 73 Orchard Drive, Kingsbridge, Devon. Have you got that?'

'Yes.' I am holding the lines in my head, repeating them to myself. *Apple, penny, table. David Barnes, 73 Orchard Drive, Kingsbridge, Devon.*

She asks me the date and I get it wrong by a day. My heart bangs harder. She asks me who the prime minister is and this I get right – though I am talking in an oddly jocose, self-conscious manner that I don't like at all. My face feels stretched.

She asks tells me to count back in sevens from a hundred. I was never quick at maths. 'Ninety-three,' I say. 'Eighty-six. Seventy-nine.' *Apple, penny, table.* 'Seventy-two.' *David Barnes.*

Next I have to give as many words as possible starting with 'P'. My mind blanks but off I shoot, hectic; my voice comes out scratchy and I am grinning foolishly. The words arrive as jerky Latinate multisyllables – *parsimonious, peri-menopausal, penitential, patriarchal, pertinacious, programmatic, plausibility* – with the occasional home-run of simple ones: *put, plant, pot, press, poppy, potato, poem.* As I reach the end of my minute, I realize I forgot all the 'ph's.

I haven't told her how I find it increasingly hard to recognize faces. I haven't told her that sometimes I'll fail to see what's in front of my eyes.

I repeat the address, and the burden of holding it in my mind lifts from me. I say: 'Apple, penny, table.' My heartbeat is slowing. She asks me to draw a clock. I do so and then see, appalled, that I've put one o'clock at midnight and midnight nowhere at all.

'You're fine,' says Claudia Wald. I know I am really, but I want to weep.

5. The Diagnosis

'We have heard the chimes at midnight.'

Leaving the memory clinic, I am slightly breathless. I feel thin-boned and insubstantial. Relief hasn't yet flowed into the place where anxiety had been; I have a sense of being scraped out. But I've been reassured that I'm still on track. Those appalling blanks, those moments of addled vacancy when I scramble around in my mind for names, dates, certainty, a sense of connectedness to the world around me, are simply a product of age and normal forgetting. I unlock my bike, put on my helmet, cycle off, the wind in my face.

However kindly and tactfully it's delivered, however parenthetical, it's a sentence. *You have dementia.* We all know that we are going to die, but we don't really know, not until we are sentenced. Dementia is a terminal illness, one that usually works with grinding slowness, chipping away at the mind's sense of itself.

'Do I use the "D" word?' asks Claudia Wald. 'It depends.'

'I felt cold water running down my spine,' says Tommy Dunne in his little bungalow in Liverpool. Beside him, Joyce sits quite upright, her face calm, her hands folded on her lap. 'I thought: "My life is over. I'll become one of those people sitting in a chair. My family will come and visit me, first once a day, then once a week, then once in months, until they don't come at all. Just me, a chair, a bed, a room."' The countdown.

Claudia Wald says that to move from fear to certainty can be a relief, and Sube Banerjee agrees. 'It can be really bad not to know. Of course, some people don't want to, but by knowing you have access to care. Knowledge is power trumps ignorance is bliss.'

But still, the sound of the gallows being built beneath the window . . .

'I take my cues from them,' Claudia tells me. 'I sometimes use euphemisms: it is possible to be honest while omitting some things. There is no simple rule: you have to respond to each person as they present themselves. I do not say: "It's a progressive, relentless disease for which there is no cure," because how many people can live with that? You have to instil as much hope as possible; make them know they are courageous to come – and they are! – and that by coming they will be supported.'

The diagnosis of dementia may be a confirmation rather than a surprise – a small step across a shifting, blurred and arbitrary line. Nothing changes and yet everything does. The person is no different the day after the diagnosis than in the days before – they are in a world that's both eerily the same and yet utterly changed and which can hold unspeakable terrors for those who are unsupported and unprepared. The bravery and endurance that the diagnosis requires – from the person who has the illness and from those who care for them – is very great. It shouldn't have to be borne alone. Often it is.

Andrew Balfour is a psychoanalytic psychotherapist and the CEO of the Tavistock Centre for Couples Relationships, where he has developed the centre's 'Living Together with Dementia' work. Both the affected individual and their partner are supported by therapeutic, person-centred interventions, particularly at the point of diagnosis, where couples can feel abandoned. He tells me of a time early in his career when he told a patient that he had dementia. He remembers watching him and his wife through the window of his room as they walked away, supporting each other, in a 'very powerful image of distress and mutual love'.

The disease crept into my father's life slowly and silently, no broken windows or alarm bells shrilling, just occasional rustles in the night, a creak on the stairs, odd things missing from their usual place but not missed. I don't know when he suspected and I don't know when we did either, or which came first. His mother had had dementia at a young age; his elder sister too. And my father had always been absent-minded – which is no indicator of dementia, but it felt like one, as if his future was woven into his benevolent, abstracted personality, the way he could disappear into his own secret world where no one could follow.

Fog thickened. His vagueness became a kind of lostness. His cheerfulness (perhaps a form of stoicism) was punctured by an anxiety that sometimes blighted his final decade, even when he was – this is one of those catch-all phrases that catches less than it drops – 'living well' with the condition.

Time heals; time undoes. In those sliding-down years there wasn't one thing, a particular event, though of course I look back now and I recognize the signs. When he struggled to remember the name of a flower that grew in the hedgerow. When his hand, holding a mug of tea, shook. When he lost his hearing aid yet again, lost track of what he was saying, lost his way (but we all do that). Scraped the car against a gateway. Left the key in the lock. When we asked him the time and he told us the cricket score (but he always was absent-minded). When on his face I would see an expression I didn't recognize (but he was always a little mysterious: he stood just out of reach). We didn't talk about it at first: when is the point at which you say, *Do you think that something is wrong, that your memory is beginning to fail you?*

There came a time when we all knew. He went to see a doctor; he had his memory test; eventually he received the sentence, hedged about with reassurances and strategies and tact, but there it was nonetheless: *you have dementia.* For me, it wasn't a punch to the solar plexus, more like a soft nudge that pushed him over that moveable line – from knowing really to really knowing. In fact, I can't even remember hearing the news.

My mother is a fighter; she believed that together they could face down the disease, hold it at bay and beat it. My father is a stoic. (Was a stoic.) He believed you must simply and with dignity endure what life hands you.

I don't know what he felt about the diagnosis. A man of inwardness and reserve, he didn't talk a great deal about his emotions and believed in getting on with things, no matter what. Up at the same time every day; make the breakfast, empty the dishwasher, mow the lawn, pay the bills, feed the birds, prune the roses, do the crossword; keep to the structure of the day, the week. That shape standing to one side, that shadow falling coldly – don't give it attention. Keep looking ahead; not too far ahead, where darkness obscures the path, just a few paces.

His role in life had been one of steady competence: he was the protector and now he needed our protection, the carer, and now he needed our care. He had looked after the finances (long after he could handle money, he kept his soft leather wallet with him and would often take it out, looking through the old membership cards that were in there), the garden, done the shopping, read the map and driven the car. (Claudia Wald tells me that, for men in particular, the issue of driving can be a watershed: 'It's a further stripping away of the self.' It's not uncommon that they refuse to take the test because of the risk of losing their licence.) He had kept the house in order, fixed things that were broken. Now something in him was broken, or breaking. To acknowledge vulnerability when his task had been to help vulnerable others was painful, almost impossible. He didn't fall apart and he didn't articulate his fears, but every so often he took to his bed, where he would lie under the covers, shaking. Life went on around him – the hum of the vacuum cleaner, the rise and fall of voices, the chink of cutlery, a phone ringing somewhere, a dog barking, cars outside, the smell of baking, of garlic frying, my mother coming softly into the room and standing beside him a while – and he would lie there until the shaking stopped.

Some people do fall apart, especially when the diagnosis comes at them like an ambush. Tommy Dunne had been told he was bipolar, and that was bad enough. But when he got lost in a car park and had a panic attack so severe that he was taken to hospital suspected of having had a heart attack, he found himself referred to an old-age psychiatrist.

'I thought, "Old-age? But I'm only fifty-seven." '

The doctor told Tommy and Joyce that the good news was that Tommy wasn't bipolar after all, and neither did he have a brain tumour. But he did have Alzheimer's. We tend to think of Alzheimer's as a memory-loss disease because, as Sube Banerjee put it, 'Memory is more measurable.' However, Tommy Dunne's particular version of the illness affects perception more than memory, is spatial as well as cognitive: 'Little bits of me feel like they've dropped off and gone missing. Everything seems nearer than it is; puddles look like gaping holes; the escalator is a chasm. Then there are gaps and jump-cuts in time. I remember being on a bus journey that I was very familiar with, had done a hundred times, and suddenly I'd missed several stops and had to get off and go back in the other direction. It was like watching things on CCTV, things jerking forward.' He smiles at me, his round face strained. 'I'm frightened of my own shadow, if I'm honest.'

Their doctor broke the news gently, telling them it was the best dementia to have and that there were many things that could be done to help him. For Joyce, it was a relief. For Tommy, it was not. He immediately imagined himself at dementia's end-stage, like one of Philip Larkin 'old fools' in his bitterly bleak poem of that name. Pessimistic, corporeal, viciously mocking but with no target to mock, the poem describes not simply anger and humiliation at old age but fear and disgust, when the mouth 'hangs open and drools' and the body disintegrates into unlovely body parts: 'Ash hair, toad hands, prune face dried into lines.' Tommy's imagined future self filled him with utter dread.

Things changed only when he and Joyce went to a post-diagnostic group and Joyce volunteered him to be part of a group working on dementia ('He gave me a stare that would have stopped a galloping horse'). Grudgingly, he went along, and once there he found that speaking out 'for my peers, the ones who don't speak', gave him confidence again. Bit by bit, he became an advocate and a spokesperson for people living with dementia: he had a purpose, a community and a status.

Tommy tells people that he meets he has dementia because he doesn't want anyone to think he's stupid. 'I'm ill, that's all.' He gets very tired (after he gives a talk he feels like he has run a marathon) and he gets very angry, and 'I grieve every day for the person I was. I miss the Tommy I used to be. But I never say, *Why me?* Why not? It's the straw I've drawn and I have to make the most of what I've got – like a torch won't work without a negative and a positive. This is the best I can make.'

Some people who get the diagnosis of dementia have already lost the capacity to understand what it is that they live with, and that lives with and inside them. They hear the words, but the words have no grip on them. Some – like Theresa Clarke – have to look at the truth full in the face ('It is what it is,' she says. 'I'm in it. I'm not embracing it and I'm not fighting it'). But as Claudia Wald acknowledges, for some it is an impossible sentence; they don't want to hear, and won't. Indeed, she believes that for several of her patients the diagnosis, however kindly delivered and appropriately supported, would be 'the death of them'. She thinks of a particular man she has recently been seeing with a 'mighty intellect' that is crumbling: she is helping and supporting him and he is on the drugs that hold back the advance of the illness, but she is not giving him that word that would topple him.

Rebecca Myers's father feared the diagnosis would topple his wife – whom he adored and fiercely protected. At the official diagnosis in 1999 she was, like Tommy, only fifty-seven. It was Rebecca – a trained nurse – who insisted that her mother needed to be properly assessed, while her father still resisted: 'He just couldn't cope. He had this terrible internal struggle: having to face something he couldn't bear to face; knowing what was coming and not knowing. He wanted to take away her struggle.'

Rebecca's mother was always terrified of the illness, having watched her own mother lost to it. Her father insisted that she should not be told the diagnosis. 'And we colluded in his decision,' says Rebecca. 'We never told her. Would it have helped her? Now, as a professional, I'd say: *How can you possibly not disclose it?* But it came from a place of love. She would ask what was wrong and we'd say, "Something's changing a bit in your brain," and she'd say, "OK. OK." The hardest bit was when she was between knowing and not knowing, going, "Why am I like this? What's the matter with me?" She started to hallucinate and they put her on meds for a while – that pharmacological cosh. She'd get up at night. Sometimes I'd arrive in the morning and find Dad in the garden, smacking his head against a tree. No one knew how to handle it. The services aren't like they are today, though the Alzheimer's Society person was fantastic. I was working part-time and looking after my two little children and trying to help Dad, but he was completely exhausted and he was grieving massively, and so I gave up work, because I couldn't bear it. And he couldn't either; he just couldn't bear to see her distressed, hallucinating, screaming. Sometimes she was frightened of him, and of me. I tried to talk to him about strategies. For instance, they used to love dancing; they went to dance halls when they were younger, and I remember how they would jive together in the kitchen. So now he would put on music and they would dance together.' She pauses; she isn't really talking to me any more. 'Theirs was a wonderful love story.'

(My parents also loved dancing, my father especially, who did a nimble foxtrot and a graceful waltz and knew how to tango. They too used to dance in the kitchen while we, embarrassed teenagers, would look away, not wanting to watch their intimacy. When they celebrated their sixtieth wedding anniversary the year before my father's wretched final year and his death, we arranged a *thé dansant* for them. It was in September, cool and blustery-bright, and we hired a little marquee for their garden. We put on an elaborate, absurd English tea – miniature cucumber sandwiches, tiny cup-cakes, éclairs cut into the shape of swans, coin-sized scones – and we set up speakers for the music they had loved in their courting days. We all wore fancy clothes, and when they were led into the garden all dressed up, she in a long red dress and he in his evening suit, we made a circle around them and they danced. Arm in arm, they danced together as the day shaded towards evening. There are things we should hold in our memories, however frail and subjective those memories may be, to set against the times of wreckage and ruin.)

For every diagnosis, half-diagnosis and diagnosis withheld, there is an avoided diagnosis: so many men and women up and down the country who, gripped by dread and humiliation, hide from their disease and in so doing hide from the world, locking themselves in with the monster they most fear.

Denial can be a valid and necessary strategy. Truth can be brutal, and we can't face up to everything. Michael Kinsley, the American political journalist and founding editor of *Slate* magazine, whose self-identity depended on 'his edge', has exuberantly defended it as a 'legitimate option'. Kinsley for many years kept his diagnosis of Parkinson's Disease secret – from other people and largely from himself, shrieking inwardly every time someone mentioned Parkinson's and cognition, *Shut up! Shut up! Shut up!* He dreaded being pitied and 'written off' and he would refuse to look at the research and the implications of his condition: 'I'll stop there, if you don't mind.' But denial is a strategy that depends on secrecy; eventually the secret springs a leak, and there often comes a time when it is no good just plugging the holes in the dyke. Truth will flood in.

There is a difference between the kind of denial we all practise and which makes the world go round and the denial that is a corrosive, self-blinding avoidance. One is a strategy to protect the vulnerable self, like a bulwark built against the storms of the world; the other is self-destructive and often agonizing. And it spreads: the area that is being desperately fenced off grows larger and larger, like a stain spreading, until everything becomes terrifying, everything taboo.

The story that Andy and Claire Bell tell me about Andy Bell's parents is one of a terrified refusal to accept dementia – a refusal that actually meant it gnawed and burrowed its way into every corner of their life, growing fat on buried secrets and lies. Before we talk – I know them already; their daughter and mine are great friends and they have been a constant, generous presence in her life – we visit Andy's mother, Jan Bell, in the home where she now lives. She is small, slightly plump; her grey hair falls around a soft, sweet face. Claire says that she was always a 'gentle, self-deprecating' presence. She is neatly dressed; her skin is smooth and she looks peaceful and content, younger than seventy-three. Her sentences are a refrain of amiability and gratitude ('I'm lucky,' she says; and 'I'm very happy'; 'Everyone is so lovely to me'; 'Oh how lucky I am'). Jan Bell believes that she is helping to run the residential home, cooking and making beds and ironing ('This is not entirely true,' says her daughter-in-law wryly) and she can be dismissive of other residents who are no longer able to talk, who wear nappies and spend their days asleep on the sofas, toothless mouths open. She blithely removes things from their rooms – teddies, soft toys: recently Claire opened her wardrobe to find a lifelike baby doll staring up at them.

It would be easy for this to be a cheerful, slightly cute story – oh, the funny things that the old get up to! But while Jan Bell might be placid and contented now, her story is full of violence. When Andy tells it to me, his shoulders are heavy and he is visibly distressed. It's the story of a marriage and of a family, for while dementia is an illness, it is one that often feeds upon the stuff of the past. Jan and her husband, Eddy, both came from poor and damaged families. At the time of their marriage, Eddy Bell was having an affair with his wife's best friend. She found out and she never forgave him. 'They loved each other; they were in their way devoted. But there was always that anger.' Perhaps in retaliation, she had an affair herself: Andy remembers walking into her bedroom while his father was working away and finding their neighbour in bed with his mother. 'She took me out of the room and told me I was having a bad dream – I didn't forgive her for that.' When his father returned, he kicked down the door of the neighbour's house and beat up the man, who was never seen again. Andy thinks that his mother had other affairs: he has memories as a child of his parents' bitter arguments, her hitting out at his father, running after him to stop him from leaving, hanging off the car as he drove away. Eddy Bell made his wife have an abortion because he didn't believe the baby was his. So there were, Andy says, understating it, 'complications and resentments in their relationship'.

When Jan Bell started forgetting things, she and her husband literally shut out the rest of the world. Although they had been sociable, they no longer went out. When Claire and Andy phoned, Eddy would prompt his wife, filling in the gaps and correcting mistakes, covering for her; they had multiple strategies for hiding the truth. Even when Eddy discovered he had all-body terminal cancer they kept the doors to their house firmly shut. Neither of them could cook any longer, and they were living on crackers; their health was rapidly deteriorating. Ashamed and terrified, they sought no help at all – not from professionals, nor from family and friends.

'As her dementia got worse, as she was increasingly remembering the distant past and was back in that time of betrayal, she –' Andy stops. 'They were in such a stressful position,' he says, looking into the distance. 'They were not coping.'

I wait. Claire waits (she knows what is coming). He looks back at us.

'She started to attack him. She would beat him up; properly beat him up. In the beginning, he could defend himself, hold her wrists to stop her, but later he couldn't. He was dying, you see. One of the reasons they couldn't ever see friends was because his arms were covered in dark bruises. I don't know when we found out. There was a Sunday lunch when we saw him covered in injuries and he told us, "Your mother did that." But he insisted we do nothing; he *insisted*.'

Claire adds: 'Jan was like a little child, looking down, walking away, not meeting our eyes. She knew what she was doing.'

'Through our lives,' says Andy, 'these terrible things happen and we put them away and don't deal with them, but Alzheimer's unlocks that door and it is open at last. She couldn't deal with her feelings then or now. Perhaps she couldn't help herself.' His body is folded over with sadness.

'It's like you put your memories in a kitchen drawer,' says Claire. 'And rattle them up and all the memories are in a sharp muddle: she remembered the feelings but not the events connected to them; she lost that connection between memory and feeling.'

Perhaps Eddy Bell wanted help but he didn't know how to ask for it. He wanted to repair the damage he had done all those years ago but knew he'd never be able to; he didn't want to be separated from her, even though they were living in torment. He hated the idea of going into a home. Then, one day, he decided to drive them both to Lake Garda, where they had had their honeymoon – 'Perhaps he thought he could jog happy memories.' He told no one. ('It was like *Thelma and*

Louise,' says Claire.) He drove there in two days. It was a terrible mistake: in that unfamiliar environment, Jan Bell was utterly disoriented, agitated and terrified. She wouldn't allow any windows to be opened and always had all the lights on. She was walking up and down, up and down, never still. They cut the holiday short and drove back again, staying for one night only. 'He was very upset, very poorly, had stopped eating anything: it was like his body was consuming itself. I went to see him and he burst into tears. My mother looked at him weeping there and just said, "What do you do with someone like that?" It was so cruel, everything was so cruel.'

The ugly disorder had to end. At last the family contacted social services and the couple went into a home together. Even there she continued to attack her husband, though she said and still says that she was looking after him. Once a carer found her dragging him out of the bed – an emaciated, dying man – and kicking him; another time, she was found wielding a bread knife, and at that point they were separated, this couple who had loved and hurt each other all their shared lives, who wanted to be together and whose only chance of peace was to be apart. Eddy Bell died soon after. Now, after time, all of Jan Bell's memories of her husband are 'nice' ones.

'I tell myself it's the illness,' Andy Bell says. 'I know it is. But she's my mother; he was my father. When I visit her and am tender, it's for him. I'm doing it for Dad.'

With Jan and Eddy Bell, dementia – undiagnosed, untreated, unsupported, hidden away in the darkness – went on the rampage. But Claudia Wald is very clear that with the right support and treatment diagnosis is the start of learning to 'live well' with the condition: 'I try to normalize it – which does *not* mean that I trivialize it. You have to gradually bring the goalposts nearer home. You have to make the most of your present and near-future.' And Sube Banerjee agrees: 'We have to focus on what the person with dementia *can* do, not what they can't. It won't be the same as it once was, and it requires time – which is the one thing we often have least of – and our ability to adapt to them, because they are not going to adapt to us. Kindness is the core. And hope. I sell hope.'

Kindness and hope. The artist Jenni Dutton is humane, upbeat and almost joyful about her mother's dementia, which has run its course now. Her mother died in 2015, five stone, blind, inarticulate, completely incontinent – 'But oh, that little soul!' says her daughter. Her face shines with memory and love.

'I saw it as the next positive step in a life,' were almost the first words that Jenni Dutton had spoken to me when we met, before seeing my surprise and adding: 'Although I'm very good at forgetting the bad bits; I always have been.'

We are sitting in the café at Salisbury Art Centre, surrounded by her 'Dementia Darnings', an extraordinary collection of sixteen tapestries that she made over the last years of her mother's life. She took photographs of her mother and squared them up on a large canvas so that she has a grid that is a guide to the placing of shapes and colour and she doesn't need to view the piece as a whole as she works, which can be a 'distraction'. So she weaves the wool, not looking at the whole image, dissociating from the nose, the mouth, the eyes, often working upside down ('A bit like having dementia,' she says – 'seeing things in patches'). The result is eerie: some of the huge portraits are lifelike and look from a distance like traditional oils; in others, the wool is pale and sparse, coming undone, and in later works it is impossible to see, close up, that this is even a picture of a face. The threads are a maze ('as is a brain') and tangled up ('like in dementia').

'I'm exploring loss,' says Jenni Dutton. 'There's such symbolism around weaving – a stitch in time, losing the thread, being like Penelope, a woman waiting. In these tapestries, things are coming apart, but it's also an act of mending.' Over the series, we see her mother recede, become less decipherable. The pictures are an account of the stages of self-loss: they depict 'one little old lady, my mum' and at the same time offer the viewer a timeless account of age and dissolution. The face is undone before our eyes, but softly, so that it feels almost like a liberation in which the stitched-up, coherent, tightly patterned self is freed into a soft unravelling. Whereas William Utermohlen scrutinized himself with a dispassionate and pitiless gaze, these images are very tender and some are so intimate it feels almost indecent to look at them. Jenni Dutton nods. 'I know. But this work is important. We mustn't shy away from decline and decay. It is crucial that we are not frightened of these vulnerable images. And my mother was supportive of my work, intrigued and proud.'

Jenni Dutton sees dementia differently from anyone else I've previously met; she views it as a difficult gift, something to be embraced rather than resisted. Her mother was very different from her – small, dainty, pretty. Her illness began gradually, but because her own mother had had dementia the family understood that she was declining. She lived in her own home and carers came in several times a day. Jenni Dutton was often there, building her working days around her mother's needs. She would ask her daughter what was wrong with her, and Jenni would reply, 'You have dementia' – but 'I always reassured her that she would be supported, and would be all right.' At the memory clinic where she received the formal diagnosis she didn't ask questions. So she both knew and did not know what was happening to her. She went slowly into the land of forgetting.

It seems that, instinctively, Jenni Dutton understood how

to accommodate the illness and enter into her mother's changed and shrinking world. If her mother rang up wanting to go to the shops and it was nine at night, 'It didn't matter.' If she ate all the food that Jenni had left out for the entire day by the middle of the morning, 'It didn't matter.' She did not come to harm, and the important thing 'was not to let her get upset'. Sometimes she would become lost and disoriented: 'She would walk and walk with her little dog; she would rattle, rattle, rattle at the doors we had to lock to keep her safe.'

In these first stages of her illness Jenni Dutton's mother was given a safe structure, boundaries ('I'm very good at boundaries myself; all those years of therapy!'), a circle of support and a form of validation. People with dementia are continually contradicted and corrected: *It's Sunday not Friday; You've already eaten your breakfast; You haven't cleaned your teeth; That vivid memory is false; I'm your wife, not your mother; I'm your daughter, not your wife; Anyway, you are old and she is dead; The past is over.* Their version of reality is denied – but reality is not a rigid structure; it's impermanent, multiple and subjective. There are many ways of seeing.

In her familiar home, with her little dog, her carers, her daughter coming several times a day, her granddaughter too, her mother managed for a while. Her life stayed pretty much on track. One day, 'we were going through photo albums and she recognized old family and friends and I started embroidering their faces on to the dress I had made: little sketches in thread.' So began a process that produced the haunting images staring down at us. It seems to me that this collaboration between mother and daughter in some strange way made the process of disintegration an exploration of loss for both of them, as well as the experience of it. They were on a poignant adventure that would end only with her mother's death.

*

According to Raymond Tallis, it is in its early stages that the illness is most eloquently expressed by the affected individual. To find the 'courage to be' in the face of the diagnosis can be painfully hard, and becomes less so only once they begin to forget. By the end, says Claudia Wald, we just have to 'pray that the fear has gone'. Shortly after William Utermohlen got his diagnosis in 1995, he made his last large painting, *Blue Skies*. In it, the artist sits alone in the empty glare of his attic studio. The walls are blue and yellow; the table is yellow; the skies are blue. The open skylight that dissects the image hangs above him like a guillotine. The slight figure sits hunched over the table, holding on to it as though it would otherwise slide away – or as though he would. Whereas the 'Conversation Pieces' are full of physical objects and the comfort of things, here there is nothing. Just a man in a space. It is a desolate, pitiless image.

'He locked himself away,' says his widow, remembering that terrible time. 'He would stare into space like one of the living dead. He was scared and he was ashamed.'

But William Utermohlen's most famous work, his revelatory self-portraiture, was ahead of him, although he did not know it (and perhaps he never knew it). When the artist was briefly admitted to the National Hospital for Neurology and Neurosurgery at Queen Square, in London, he met the nurse Ron Isaacs. It was Isaacs who encouraged him to continue drawing and to portray himself. So he picked up his brush once more. Painting and drawing were the ways in which he could connect his inner self to the outer world; they gave him his voice, the thread that would take him out of the labyrinths of the self. For a while . . .

6. Shame

'Pray, do not mock me: I am a very foolish fond old man . . .
Do not laugh at me.'

Most of us find it extremely painful to be laughed at, to be the
joke in the room. Perhaps it is even more distressing to people
of my father's generation, for whom dignity is central to their
notion of identity. And I think men are often more wounded
by the loss of dignity than women.

When I look back at the early stages of my father's dementia
and try to imagine what it must have been like for him during
those early years, I slide up against something soft, insidious.
Not loss (though loss is there), not fear (although that too), or
denial (of course), or a sense of life continuing after all (I hope)
and the comfort of ordinary moments. Something else. A sen-
sation that makes the skin prickle and the guts coil: doors
flung open, eyes watching, lights switched on in the darkness
and if you cover your face your naked body is exposed; the
sound of knowing laughter and the intake of breath. Layer
after protective layer is pulled away, the defences that have
been built up over a lifetime crumble, and something pulpy
and secret and infinitely vulnerable, something that no one
should ever see, even those who love you most, especially
those who love you most, is laid bare.

My father sometimes pulled the covers over his head and
lay in the darkness, wrapped in his own warmth where no one

could see him. He didn't exactly hide his diagnosis, but nor did he talk about it. By some kind of unspoken agreement, we didn't use the 'D' word to him. His friends skirted around it.

Jan and Eddy Bell pulled the door shut, *click*, locked it against the world. Tommy Dunne closed the curtains, turned out the light, unplugged the phone. Patricia Utermohlen says her husband would sit alone in his studio; he was scared and above all he was 'ashamed'.

Shame is a word that comes up over and over again in connection with dementia. I spoke recently to someone whose father would not – could not – tell anyone of his diagnosis of early-onset dementia even though that had meant losing his job and his livelihood. I know of many couples who tell nobody – although, of course, lots of people know or guess and, of course, the couple knows that they know . . . But it's a secret; a dirty secret; shameful.

Almost everyone I have talked to whose lives have been personally touched by the illness has spoken about their sense of shame. Shame comes in many guises and is felt by the affected individual and, by association, their family. Shame because of the stigma; shame because of the loss of power and control; shame because identity is cruelly stripped away and leaves the vulnerable self exposed; shame because, over time, the disease becomes so bodily and the body is a messy, leaking vessel; shame at the acute loss of dignity; shame because the person with dementia feels repeatedly caught out; shame because bit by bit all those things that have been kept private and hidden are on display; shame because we are all performative beings and learn to act out our selves on the stage of our lives, but dementia brings the mortification that comes in our dreams of standing in front of an audience and not remembering our lines, of being found sitting on a toilet with everyone watching, of being seen naked. Naked in our body and in our soul: that soft and quivering part of us that we try all our lives to protect from the judging world – and, crucially, from ourselves.

When people talk of the shame caused by dementia, it is often deeply connected to the failing body. It's about *mess*. While other things spill out – obscenities, mumbles, cries, wild and garbled speech, an incoherent flow of the mind that's lost hold of itself – it's the physical manifestations of loss of control that can be the most upsetting and humiliating. We learn from a very young age to keep things in or to let them out only in private: the incontinent waste of the self. The inside comes out in unwanted ways when the boundaries that have been policed for so long and with such rigour collapse. 'Don't worry; it's natural; it's just your body,' I hear a nurse say reassuringly to a patient. But a body is never *just* a body. A body is where we live and how we live.

And there is in dementia an additional terror about what has occurred during those periods that are erased from memory, leaving only an indistinct imprint of disquiet, the nudge beneath the ribs. Something happened. What happened? What did I do and what did people see? Was it ridiculous? Was *I* ridiculous?

I have a vivid un-memory from when I was about sixteen. I went to visit my elder sister, who was at a university in Devon and sharing a house with a group of friends. I was anxious not to let her down and I wanted to impress her friends; I wanted them to like me. There was a small party in their house and I drank a large amount of cheap, harsh cider. I got hideously drunk. I have no idea what I did, what I said, where I went. It's an unforgiving blank into which excruciating fragments drift: me in the toilet with one of those young men who I wanted to impress holding back my sticky hair; me lying in bed with my sister sitting beside me, being kind; me wandering around the garden, holding forth about poetry or love or something; me weeping about a relationship that was going awry. The next morning, feeling grimly awful and embarrassed, I went to the sea with my sister. We didn't speak about the night before; I tried to behave as if nothing had happened. It was very sunny and I lay on a rock, slack and nauseous, and slept. When I woke I still felt awful but now I was sunburnt as well, hot and stinging and rawly scarlet. It was as if my face wore a perma- nent blush of shame. I kept seeing myself as I might have been during those awful lacunae: I imagined what I must have looked like when I had no control over how I presented myself to the world, how risible. Even now, decades later, a wash of remembered humiliation passes through me.

A sense of shame is an essential part of being a self-conscious individual and having an identity; it lives in the gap between the self's actions and its standards. People with no shame at all and therefore no self-censorship may violate the notion of what it is to be a social, decent being. But shame, with its sense of being watched and judged, can bring a toxic self-consciousness.

The self as other, the self met in the mirror, the self naked in the world and the sense of flooding shame – not at anything done or said or thought or imagined, no flushing out of secrets, but shame without a useful object. The self as the object of shame. Patricia Utermohlen used to have to cover up mirrors because her husband was so terrified of seeing himself exposed in them: he had become unbearable to himself, an object of acute humiliation. Quite often, in hospitals or homes, I see people with dementia put their hands over their faces, hiding in plain sight from a world of shame.

*

Dementia is pitiless. It unpicks not just the sense of self but the control over that self. My father was never vain, but he did care about how he presented himself to the world. He shaved every morning without fail (and probably didn't look deliberately in the mirror for the rest of the day); he polished his shoes and tied the laces with a firm double bow; he combed his hair, tucked in his shirt; when he went to work it was in a nice suit with the tie done up just so. Even when he was alone, he never 'let himself go' (I let myself go all the time). He used to say that 'a gentleman is someone who uses his butter knife in private' – and we'd hoot with laughter and mock him, because who talks about gentlemen and who has a butter knife? But I think he would have used his butter knife in private if he'd had one, and would have shaved on a desert island, and polished his shoes. Because you keep up appearances – and this isn't a shallow thing at all, it's rooted in the sense of self. Shame assaults that self-image.

In the early years of his illness he would have vivid false memories, not uncommon in dementia. They were almost always connected with public humiliation: the one that repeated most often was to do with driving, or no longer being allowed to drive. He thought – remembered – that he had been in his car and police on motorbikes were following him, their faces concealed by helmets and visors, horribly impersonal forces of the law. It was like something out of Kafka's *The Trial*. They pulled him over and told him he had been driving dangerously and took away his licence (which had indeed been taken away from him). In frequent versions of this paranoid story his name was given to the newspapers so that everyone could read of his failure – which was a failure of male competence. He would write formal, distressed letters to the council trying to clear his name, which had been dishonoured.

People who live with dementia need more than ever to be treated with respect and dignity; it's a fragile carapace that protects the vulnerable and terrified self. Often, of course, the opposite happens: they become objects of mockery. When Rita Hayworth was in her first stages of dementia people thought she was drunk and ridiculed her. As they did the Prime Minister Harold Wilson. And President Reagan. And Margaret Thatcher, looking vague and clutching at her handbag in her later years (she was known to be partial to whisky). People with dementia are often laughed at, because forgetting oneself is perilously close to the stuff of farce: the clothes put on clownishly askew or not put on at all, the garbled sentences that can be a source of hilarity, the muddle over dates and times, the mistaken identities, the sudden obscenities, all the banana skins and all the slip-ups. But the joke's on them; the joke *is* them. 'Pray do not mock me,' says King Lear, as his patriarchal, self-aggrandizing identity is dismantled and he is at last left as a bare, forked worm, a human among other humans. 'I am a very foolish fond old man.' In Ian McKellen's revelatory portrayal of Lear, he took off all his clothes and stood before us, an old man whose descent into madness was a form of dementia and whose nakedness was of the soul as well as the body.

I can hardly bear to think of my father, my courteous, proud father who polished his shoes every day, shaved carefully, knotted his tie just so, washed his hands like a surgeon about to perform an operation, being ashamed.

Sitting in Theresa Clarke's little living room in her bungalow in Antrim, I ask her – with some trepidation – if she ever feels ashamed. She puts her head to one side. 'Ashamed?'

'Yes.'

'Nicci,' she says, as if she is a bit disappointed in me. I should know her better. 'We've got to know what makes us tick. If we don't, we're losing ourselves, dementia or not. You have to delve into yourself. I feel that I know the real me. I feel no shame because I can't be caught out.'

Not many of us can't be caught out.

Shame. Humiliation. Exposure. I used to think that guilt was the superior emotion – the voice of conscience, inner-directed, the 'sound in oneself of the voice of judgement' – whereas shame seemed more narcissistic, a kind of superficial vanity and petty sense of mortification; that blushing, flushing, sometimes crippling adolescent self-consciousness. I thought that as one became more confident and wise (oh, if only) then shame would fall away and the deeper, less egotistic sense of guilt would take its place as the pilot of behaviour. But shame, though connected with appearance, is an enduring and deep-rooted human emotion.

'Identity and shame are intimately connected,' says Gerard de Vries in Utrecht. 'You become an ego by building up a self-consciousness, and that brings shame.' It's not just decorum or prudishness or embarrassment. A 'crucial part of self-respect is respect in the eyes of others', and this need has deeper roots than rationality or self-determination: respect is intimately related to shame and 'both are inseparable from one's identity and visibility in the social order'. Shame is the shame of one-self before the other – it's a defiling exposure and a kind of appalling recognition that I am as the other sees me. Shame is the shame of the self. I am that object.

In *Shame and Necessity*, the philosopher Bernard Williams discusses the implications of the inner world coming up against the outer one. The basic experience connected with shame, he writes, is 'that of being seen, inappropriately, by the wrong people, in the wrong condition. It is straightforwardly associated with nakedness.' (The roots of the words 'shame' and 'genitals' are apparently indistinguishable in many languages.) Where guilt is rooted in hearing – the voice of judgement and condemnation – shame is rooted in sight and in nudity. It always involves the gaze of another, but it can be an imagined gaze of an imagined other: the internalized other; the respected, ethical other. So it can mean the exposure of the self by the self; the disclosure of the self to the self. And it happens at a much deeper level than egotism and the failure to live up to other people's expectations. In its experience, one's whole being seems diminished: 'The other sees all of me, and all through me, even if the occasion for shame is on the surface, for instance in my appearance; and the expression of shame . . . is not just the desire to hide, or hide my face, but to disappear.' To disappear: to cover one's face, to hide one's head in one's hands, to want to crawl into a hole, to sink into the ground; to wish the ground would swallow one up. *I could have died.*

'The contradiction between inner and outer' which Helen Small identifies in her humane and wide-ranging book exploring old age, is 'of a different order to anything we have previously faced.' This is powerfully amplified in the early stages of dementia. The self watches the self that declines, is both the subject and the object, the cringing audience and the actor who keeps forgetting their lines, whose soiled trousers are around their ankles, who stumbles through the wrong door into the wrong room and on whose face is a look of humiliated surprise. To see your self as a disgraced other; to see your face in the glass but it belongs to your dead father, or to a disgraced interloper failing to perform the self you spent so long making.

⋆

At the Tavistock Centre, psychoanalysts Tim Dartington and Andrew Cooper and Claire Kent, clinical lecturer in social work, talk to me about 'confabulation' – which means, says Andrew Cooper, 'enacting a pretence'. People with dementia often find *alibis* for themselves, says Tim Dartington (whose wife, Anne, died with dementia at an early age and who herself wrote eloquently about the disease that came upon her slowly, like a fox, and about her 'unfaithful brain'). 'But,' he goes on, 'you give yourself away by continually repeating it, getting it slightly wrong. We want to be found but not found out – and some people with dementia devote large amounts of energy to avoiding discovery: not just literally hiding away but finding strategies that will cover up memory lapses, confusions and mistakes.'

Alongside the alibis that Tim Dartington talks of there's the habit of generalizing: asking questions or making comments that do not disclose lack of knowledge. It may be that the person with dementia does not know if they are seeing you for the first time in months or have seen you a few minutes ago and are trying to gauge this with their vague greeting. It may be that they know that they know you but are not quite sure of the exact relationship and are looking for cues. Or that they remember that they've been asked to do something but can't remember what. It's hard and stressful work to be continually ad-libbing, catching hold of prompts, finding landmarks, small patches of solid ground amid swampy uncertainty.

People who care for the person who has dementia – above all, if they are their partner or spouse and have built up a relationship of mutual affirmation – often collaborate with them in this task of confabulation. After all, they have been taking part in the same performance for so long, a double act and each other's audience. Just as Eddy Bell prompted his wife in terror that she would reveal their shared secret, so carers give their loved ones alibis, cover for them, finish their sentences, take up the stories they are telling, explain them to others, even join in with the stressful pretence of normality.

In part this is a simple act of kindness: if shame springs from the understanding that the vulnerable inner self needs protection, then of course you will help someone you love with this act of protection. But because in relationships the identity of the other and the self are bound together, more or less tightly, shame can spread from one to the other like an intimate contagion. We do not just suffer and grow anxious with the other but within ourselves, because where does one person end and the other begin? When people recoil and keep their distance, it may not be because they lack compassion and empathy but because they feel so endangered.

'Yes indeed,' says Pat Utermohlen stoutly. She is determined not to shy away from full disclosure and she wants other people to know that their feelings of shame are not shameful. 'I certainly did feel shame sometimes. He would defecate in the most inconvenient places. There was a time at Kew Gardens. It was a nightmare. I was very embarrassed – there I was on the train with this smelly creature. Or arriving at a friend's house and he would defecate.' She nods. 'But I always took him with me. I am not squeamish. But it's very hard.'

The shame that the person with dementia feels largely belongs to the earlier stages of dementia. That it often falls away during later stages, when the body fails and the narrative self is dismantled, is one of the few kind losses amid a pile-up of cruel ones. They no longer know – or if they know, they don't care – that they wear a nappy, defecate, urinate, dribble, make sounds that are not intelligible. They have returned to a state of innocence, before the fall into self-consciousness and identity.

In *Out of Mind* by J. Bernlef, the saddest and most illuminating work of fiction about the illness that I've read, his narrator Maarten is at first aware of this dislocation and is in a state of constant anxiety and hyper-alertness. He sees people look at each other when he is speaking; he knows when he puts a foot wrong and tries to retreat to a place of safety. He understands the importance of holding on to routine events or, when that fails, to imitate them: 'To lie and then believe the lie – to invent a life from minute to minute.' Bit by bit he loses his tormenting sense of wrongness. When he utters obscenities, he feels no responsibility. When he touches himself in the bath, giving himself an erection, he can't understand the horrified reaction of the nurse and his wife. When he sees an old man in the mirror, his 'belly streaked with shit', he is glad that it isn't him.

When eventually the memory and the relationships that have held the self together dissipate, then the individual is adrift between self and other, times and places, night and day. While for an observer this may be uniquely terrifying, there can be a kind of mercy that oblivion delivers – the kindness of letting the bewildered, frantic, humiliated self go. To no longer recognize oneself; to no longer feel panic and shame. To be in the world and not distinct from it.

But the shame they have mercifully been released from can be passed to those who look after them. For carers, particularly partners and spouses, it is often hard or impossible to rid themselves of a sense of inherited humiliation. In a relationship that has lasted decades, the boundaries between self and other are blurred and identification is intimately bound up with the other. If they become the voices and the memory of the person with dementia, why not the shame as well?

This shame goes deeper than humiliation and the fear of being seen naked and defiled: it becomes existential, spreading through the whole of society, and it is one of the reasons we have dealt so inadequately with dementia as a disease. In the breached and self-forgetful state of those who are living and dying with the condition, we recognize our once and future selves. We want to resist identification. The squeamishness and horror that the spectacle of a person with advanced dementia can provoke comes not just from the way the disease, at its most cruel, dismantles a person, leaving them demolished and yet still alive. It threatens us by dismantling our sense of our own selfhood and predicts our future disgrace. One day, I may be like that. One day, I may wear a nappy, be turned in my bed and washed, shout long-kept secrets to the world. It's hardly bearable; we turn away so that we do not have to bear it. Society turns away. Not me, not us, but *them*: the disgraced other.

Jenni Dutton's tender, unsqueamish, entirely accepting relationship with her mother during her long dementia years has much to teach us as a society. Somehow, she found the wisdom and humanity to look steadfastly at what it is to be a failing mind inside a wasting body and feel nothing but compassion, love and joy. Indeed, she seemed to be able to see her mother more clearly and value her more dearly as capacity fell away. She didn't mourn what she had lost but embraced what she had become: 'That little soul!'

Yet this avid shame – which spies at us through keyholes and sniggers from corners – is also crucial to society as a whole. It's like a law enforcer that keeps us on track emotionally, psychologically, socially, politically and morally. Civilization is held together by shame far more than by guilt. Good behaviour is maintained by it; rules are followed and promises are kept because of it; politicians rise and fall by it; morality is upheld in the knowledge that we watch and we are watched. Shame keeps an eye on us and holds us to account.

In *The Republic*, Plato considers the question posed by the Ring of Gyges, a mythical object which makes its owner invisible at will (a bit like the one in Tolkien's *Lord of the Rings*): what would we do if no one could see us doing it? People who care for those with dementia, especially in its later stages, wear the Ring of Gyges a lot of the time. The one person who can see and feel what they are doing will forget it. Nobody will know – except for the watching self, the *I* that observes the *I*. Dementia often does its work in secret, behind closed doors. It is impossible to know how much abuse goes on in homes, in hospitals, in care homes, in any place where powerless people are unable to say what is being done to them. In the US, the National Council on Ageing recently reported that nearly half of people living with dementia experienced abuse or neglect – this includes physical and emotional abuse, confinement, passive neglect, wilful deprivation and financial exploitation. Carers often say that their loved ones are not treated with dignity while in hospital. Stories about abuse in care homes are grimly familiar. I don't think that bad people are doing bad things but that good people are – because the work is hard, stressful, underpaid, undervalued and because no one is watching and they have failed to watch themselves. If they did watch themselves, how would they bear it? Shame is useful.

In the domestic home, the person who looks after the person with dementia usually works alone. It's a hard task, both physically and emotionally, and can become hellish. Where there was once reciprocity, now less and less comes back. The person who hears what you are saying is you. The person who sees what you are doing is you. If you don't watch yourself, who knows what will happen (what does happen)?

When my father was in his middle stage of forgetfulness I remember occasionally feeling an odd, unsettling self-consciousness when I was alone with him. It was like I was in an echo-chamber, my voice coming back at me. I was aware that I was talking to him a bit artificially sometimes, as if I were performing the part of someone being nice to their father who had dementia. And I was. Because my father no longer responded in the way that he used to, I was standing in for him as well, becoming my own audience. Being a daughter and acting a daughter; talking to my father and talking to myself.

Disie Johnson, a friend of Pat Utermohlen who often joins us for our talks because her husband also has dementia, writes me an email before one meeting that reminds me of what I used to feel. 'Living with someone with dementia who is not making much sense out of life and struggles to comprehend simple things is like having to act a part all the time . . . I have to pretend that it's perfectly normal to lead this life of conversation – if I can even use that word – that is really just a series of requests by me, or repetitions of what I've just said, or explanations . . . being with a person with dementia all the time is a bit like being on stage all the time, or at least acting a part all the time, and perhaps this is why we get so tired.' She goes on: 'And all the while, in very, very slow motion, you are watching the disintegration of a person in the real sense of *person*.' When we meet that evening she talks about this sense of her own theatricality: 'Such self-control!' Her laugh is wry. 'Such a fine performance. I'm looking at myself and asking: *How are you doing? How are you reacting? Are you being good?* I try to be good. I'm lucky that he is so very sweet.' She's not sweet: she's sour, dry, splendid, theatrical and authentic, acting herself out in the theatre of her life.

7. The Carers

'How far that little candle throws his beam.'

And so, enter the carer, the caregiver – who has of course been on stage all along, just not noticed.

The story of dementia is also the story of those who care for people living with the illness. And if people with dementia are missing people, so too are their carers. In the UK, one in eight adults are carers (that's 6.5 million people), and almost 60 per cent of these are women. They save the economy an estimated £132 billion a year – and yet the carer's allowance is currently £62.10 for a minimum thirty-five-hour week: £1.77 an hour (at the time of writing, the national minimum wage is £6.70 an hour). They are undervalued and largely unrecognized, but without them the structures of society would collapse.

The carers of people living with dementia make up a large portion of this vast, invisible army: in the UK, about 700,000 men and women look after people with dementia (in the US, there are about 43.5 million carers, 15.7 million of whom look after someone with dementia). Sixty to seventy per cent of them are women; the longer the caring lasts, the higher the percentage of them are likely to be women – in other words, women carers tend to have more endurance in this hardest of tasks. Forty-four per cent of carers have a long-standing illness or disability, including depression; many of them are partners or spouses and are therefore likely to be older themselves; in the US, the average age of a female family carer of someone with dementia is 69.4. Thirty per cent of those caring have been doing so for between five and ten years, and just over 20 per cent for over ten years. In the UK in 2013, an estimated 150,000 years were spent caring for people with dementia, or 1,340 million hours.

My mother never had to become my father's 'carer'. She remained his wife, living with him and loving him as he inched towards self-loss. In the final, terrible year she could not possibly have looked after him: she was in her eighties, disabled by years of chronic back injuries and registered blind. A rota of professionals came in to do the jobs (lifting, cleaning, dressing and undressing . . .) that are so bodily and for many intimate carers so distressing. So, by and large, she remained his wife, and he her husband. She was lucky in this.

'It's a killer,' a friend who cares for her husband says to me. 'It's *savage*.'

To care. To be careful, never careless or carefree. To be care-worn. To be a carer.

We say it easily, indiscriminately, carelessly. 'Carer' is a word in whose small frame lives a great jostle of seething emotions, an army of feelings that collide and clash, while all the time the image is one of saintliness, a serene self-sacrifice in the name of duty and affection. In the same way, the word 'caregiver' has a troubling ambiguity about it. It makes care seem like an object rather than a process, and it presents the act of caring as a gift, something one person generously and self-sacrificially offers and the other receives, implying a lack of reciprocity. Some people prefer the careful new term of 'care partner'.

It matters what words we use. Vocabulary is always active. To 'accompany' someone on their journey into loss and into darkness: can we ever really do this? To be the 'loved one' when sometimes the loved one doesn't feel love at all but hostility, alienation, abandonment, repugnance and despair.

Because dementia happens in slow motion it is barely possible to say at what point the term 'carer' sticks. A woman who has been a wife for fifty years (or of course the man who has been a husband), whose husband is perhaps the only lover she has ever had, finds herself taking on the tasks that used to be his, making decisions he used to make, taking over the finances, covering up for his slips. She finds herself becoming the diary-keeper, reminding him of where he is supposed to be. The timekeeper. She stops him getting lost, or finds him when he is. She comforts him when he is anxious. She tries not to become impatient when he repeats himself – or shows her impatience and then feels guilty. She tries to remember that it is the illness not the man when he shouts at her or is indifferent and cold. She tries not to mind that what she does, day in and day out, is unseen, unvalued: nobody to say thank you or tell her she is doing a good job. She tries not to resent the fact that she is giving up things for a person who doesn't understand her self-relinquishment. She tries to hold on to her own self but feels it is slipping away from her and that life is unfair. And so it goes, slowly, slowly, a gradual incremental loss, until one day she finds that he no longer remembers what happened yesterday or that morning; he can't recall things they did together; their shared memory bank is dwindling away; their relationship is no longer one of reciprocity. She is the memory, the voice, the judgement, the choice, the custodian of their past, the narrator of their story, the gatekeeper. Then she is talking to him very patiently like he is a child – or loudly and crossly, like he is a very naughty child; she is helping him eat; she is feeding him like he was a baby; then she is washing him, then she is wiping his bottom, then she is clearing up the mess and trying not to feel disgust. This body she once desired. Then she is putting on his nappy, sleeping in a different bed. Then he is shouting at her, attacking her with shit-encrusted nails. Then he calls her 'Mummy'. Then he has no name for her. He has no words. He is a figure in a bed. She finds she is alone and everything they made together has crumbled about her, a wreckage of the future.

At what point in this inching towards obliteration does she become the 'carer'? At what point does the child who is looking after the parent call themselves 'carer' – and how do they accommodate the wrenching, dislocating experience of seeing their mother, their father, so helpless, so very bodily. Some people talk of the hard privilege of being a carer: Tim Dartington, who looked after his wife, Anne, and kept her at home during her last years, told me that what happened with his wife 'transformed my whole way of thinking, who I was, what I was doing, what my values were. It changed everything. I was a better person for it . . .' Ronnie Carroll, a dear friend of William Utermohlen who was steadfast during his last terrible years and cared for him tirelessly, spoke with tenderness and love about the experience in the short film made about the artist: 'Poor Bill got really bad. I would give him a shave; if he needed to go to the toilet, take him to the toilet. I'd make him lunch – he was a great eater; he loved eating, especially if there was a chocolate ice at the end of it . . . Then I'd get him dressed . . . and we'd go out, along the canal . . . to his favourite pub, and we'd sit and have a couple of half-lagers and we'd tell these silly stories and laugh. It was magical. It was the closest bond I've ever had with a man in my whole existence. It made me a different person, there's no doubt about it.'

But other people speak of the despair and the erosion of

selfhood. Andrew Cooper at the Tavistock Centre tells me of a patient he had when he was a social worker whose way of life was 'unsustainable' and who could no longer make any decisions for herself: 'It's the most anxiety I've almost ever felt, in my entire life. It was a void. The void was in her and in us. There was nothing to connect to and I felt panic, which probably reflected the panic in her' – but he was a professional and could go home at the end of the day.

'She has possessed me and I am diminished,' writes Andrea Gillies in her excruciating memoir about her mother-in-law, *Keeper*.

Caring can be exhausting, farcical, revelatory, horrifying, enriching, tragic. In the act, the physical and the emotional fuse. People find themselves, lose themselves; give things up and take things on; are diminished and expanded; behave terribly and beautifully; are proud of themselves and ashamed; never do well enough and do more than could possibly be expected of them. 'Carer': there should be another word.

The word 'selfless' is almost always used as a term of praise: the voluntary abandonment of one's own wishes and desires for the sake of another. I've read a large number of books in the past year that speak of the act of selfless care in rapturous and almost religious or spiritual terms. Whereas curing is directed towards recovery and has a high value in society, caring is an end in itself. One writer compares this to the myth of heroic Prometheus (the Titan who defied the gods and was punished by them when he gave the human race the gift of fire) and stoic Sisyphus (who in Hades was condemned to repeatedly roll a rock up a hill, only to see it roll down once more).

In a utilitarian sense, caring has little value and should be thought of in the light of a 'covenant' and 'fidelity'. Reciprocity may be limited or even, in dementia's end stages, entirely absent, and often achievements lie in what is *not* seen: no bedsores, no malnutrition, no falls . . . The carer needs to find meaning in the act itself, regardless of any outcome, regardless of any recognition. They are the 'keeper of the psyche' and must be a 'person of faith'. The writer and professor of nursing Sally Gadow believes that caring is the process of entering another's vulnerability and brokenness and 'breaking oneself'. In this mutual brokenness, acts that are thought demeaning in a cure model (like lifting, washing and feeding) become 'bonds of the covenant'.

This is pure selflessness: to enter into the other's word of fear and loss and frailty; to leave your own world behind; to leave your own *self* behind in order to accompany the one who is in need. It places a high value on self-relinquishment and suffering. While such a way of thinking about the act of care recognizes the profundity of the task and places unquantifiable value upon it, it at the same time attacks the notion of autonomy, independence and selfhood. Well, of course, 'autonomy' is too easy a word, as is 'agency'; all these phrases I have so blithely thrown around throughout my adult life – standing my own ground, being my own self. Is there ever such an untrammelled thing? We are born into dependency and dependency is part of the human condition. In the journey through life, our experience as flesh and blood, as a self with a body, an embodied mind, as a part of a rich and changing network of relationships, is one of continual vulnerability. Perhaps our twenty-first-century world has become too preoccupied with defences and with boundaries. Boundaries must always be breached. Caring for others and being cared for in our turn is part of the fabric of civilization. The most basic questions about how to live a good life are questions of relations. We are all connected politically, emotionally, psychologically. And yet, and yet . . .

To be selfless necessarily means not be in relationship to others (because, without self, there can be no reciprocal relationship), so how is it that women, in particular, have come to speak of themselves as if they didn't have a voice or experience desire? Carol Gilligan, the American ethicist, feminist and psychologist and author of the classic work *In a Different Voice*, explores how hero legends such as *The Iliad* or *The Odyssey* are tales of radical separation; they are the exemplary stories for men, tracing an individual drama of separation, the dream to which relationships are subordinate. All the while Penelope sits patiently at home, waiting, weaving, remembering and holding faith. Masculinity, Gilligan argues, has long been defined through separation, femininity through attachment. But how much empathy should women and all those in nurturing and 'female' roles be expected to have? Should they be destroyed by it?

Unconditional love – the greatest of gifts – is ravaging. Many parents know this with their children, for whom they would lay down their lives without pause. When I became a mother (each time I became a mother), I was shattered by the rush of rapturous, self-obliterating devotion to this little creature, pink and bawling and new, who was utterly dependent on me. I put up no resistance at all. I used to say I fell in love, plummeted; but I also felt lifted out of the tangle of myself into a pure and dangerous realm where all my energies were directed towards this tiny, powerful, endlessly demanding, tyrannical other. Motherhood can be a category that swallows up all the other selves. It's seductively easy to get lost in it because love for a child is so absorbing and unanswerable. And it's painfully hard to rescue oneself from being secondary, invisible, self-sacrificial, adoring, mythical; from being annihilated as a person who has desires, craves freedom (and sleep), wants to be foolish and irresponsible and childish.

But in this consuming love story babies become children become teenagers become adults, grow up and grow away and leave home, and you release each other. The tide that rushed in ebbs out. Love doesn't abate but the nature of the attachment changes. For carers of those with dementia, when the self is being unmade rather than made, the flow is all in the opposite direction, towards helplessness and diminishment. Leaving home is dying.

The philosopher Jane English poses the question 'What do children owe their parents?' And she answers, like a hammer coming down: 'Nothing.' In her view, parental love and sacrifice do not create debts, rather they create love and friendship: filial obligation can serve as a 'maleficent ideological warrant for the destruction of daughters'. Like Persephone locked into darkness, there is a mysterious disappearance of the female self into the underworld. If I think of my own children, then I pretty much agree with Jane English: they owe me nothing. There are no debts and there should be no guilt. They should be free of me. And yet it doesn't work the other way round: I do feel I owe a great deal to my parents and would be crippled by guilt if I didn't in some way try to repay them for all they did for me. It's not only love, it is a sense of obligation and perhaps it is also a sense of self-respect. I have an image of the person that I want to be.

But history is full of unseen, silenced women – silenced in the name of love.

'Everyone gets it for kids,' says Sube Banerjee. 'As a parent, you will compromise in what you believe, not just what you do. But our generation finds it difficult to make the same kind of compromises for our parents. There is a pleasure that comes from realizing what you are doing is pleasurable for the other person – that instead of them failing at things, you are enabling them to succeed. It's true that the traditional notion of autonomy is exploded; you have to trade off things like success, and that's really complicated. Kindness is the core,' he adds. 'And the state doesn't provide kindness; it can't. It's our problem, and there are things one gives and takes as one goes through the stages of loss.'

For surely the endeavour – the never-quite-possible endeavour – for a carer is to tread the quicksand strip of middle ground between the abandonment of the self in the name of love and duty and the unyielding protection of the self in the name of survival. To both give and keep hold of the self, to accompany the person who is leaving while also staying behind. To have courage, stamina, compassion, empathy, to be in it for the long haul and yet not to be wrecked to the point of self-extinction. If selflessness is the ideal and the aim, if suffering is seen as a virtue in itself, the carers – those hundreds of thousands of people up and down the country, those millions across the world, who, unseen and undervalued, toil at their Sisyphean task in the name of duty and of love – will always feel that their work is never good enough. Guilt floods in – guilt at being human and having desires and needs of one's own. Health and survival can come to seem like acts of infidelity; to have a space for oneself a betrayal.

In 2017, I talked to two women who have meant a great deal to me, in their different ways. The first, Mary Jacobus, was once my tutor. She was still young when I was an undergraduate and I was both a bit scared of her (although she isn't a scary woman but softly spoken and attentive) and wanted to be her. She was – and still is – attractive, quite private, formidably clever, scrupulous, self-questioning and kind; a woman of integrity. She was a bit of a pin-up for the male students: I remember her giving her lectures sitting on the edge of the platform, wearing boots. (And because I had been brought up to be a good girl, I also vividly remember an occasion when, in a small seminar when I was the only woman, she asked who would drink their coffee out of a jam jar, since she had run out of mugs, and I at once offered. She looked at me severely: 'No. I'm asking the men. Don't do that.' A small jolt of pleasure ran through me.)

We didn't lose touch. I have visited Mary and her husband in Ithaca, upstate New York, when her children were little and sat in her lovely old house there, full of books and paintings and baby clothes (she has lived there for four decades but is now in the process of selling and 'dismantling', downsizing to a condo); been to her terraced house in Cambridge when she was living there; she has come to see me, bearing a fragrant rose bush that still stands in my garden. She's become my friend – my friend whose husband has dementia. He was diagnosed several years ago and is now entering the mid-stage of the illness, and she is his main carer – although 'carer' is a world she has grave reservations about. Throughout her career, she has been a powerful advocate for women's writing and the female voice. She's a feminist who came of age in its second wave, and she is psychologically acute about the ways in which women have to actively resist selflessness: the ideal of female saintliness that can be deadly. She talks about the experience carefully, without resentment or self-pity; she's her own shrewdest critic. She is experiencing it and she is thinking about it, what it means, how to find a way to live, what her boundaries should be. She is thinking about how to survive.

Normality, she tells me, provides a form of scaffolding: they walk their dog each day (an adopted border collie who is a great bond); they do, or try to do or fail to do, the *Guardian* crossword together. But 'it is endlessly difficult to do or think about anything other than managing our situation in Ithaca day by day . . . it consumes all the time unless I absent myself.'

'It's a two-body problem,' she says to me as we sit in the café of the Fitzwilliam Museum in Cambridge. 'My own mind is affected. I'm not just the memory. I'm also the anxiety.'

Her husband has become 'happy-go-lucky. He doesn't recognize his limits. So I have to be the anxious one.' Because he feels omnipotent, he can experience any kind of criticism as a form of persecution, a 'very primitive thing'. She becomes his 'corrector'. She also becomes a kind of narrator for him, making order out of what is confused, foggy and 'in pieces'. This is a difficult enterprise, one that threatens the balance of her life. 'You have to keep time for yourself,' she says. 'One needs to defend oneself, to preserve one's own mind. Where there is chaos, you have to manage it. Splitting is a kind of defending. I've always been quite fierce – and maybe frightened of being dependent; of being powerless and helpless.' She adds: 'Carers go on and on and on and on.'

She went to a course that promised 'powerful tools' that would help carers – and it turned out that really the most powerful tool was simply: 'Do something for yourself, every day.' The thing that she chooses to do for herself is to go to the library. She also goes to an Italian class and she continues to write, although the hours that belong to her are increasingly rare. 'But sometimes, when I walk out of the door, I feel as if I'm handing Reeve over: "You take over, Nanny." That doesn't feel good. But if I didn't do it, I'd be wholly absorbed in that world. And I mustn't be.'

Her father had dementia at the end of his life. He was a 'very difficult man, and his dementia made him more so'. Her mother had a terrible time of it and then she 'dumped' him in a home. 'The cruelty was desperation. She was trying to save her own life. I don't ever want to become so desperate that I would be cruel like that.'

So she acts with care and thought, is not reckless or self-destructive, trying against the grain of her character to be patient, trying always to be kind although acutely aware of the frustrations and the diminishing returns of intimacy. She is making sure her commitment is sustainable and durable, portioning out her time and her energy. 'And I still have him. My loss is not a mourning so much as a letting go – of the past, of opportunities. It's very painful. Now I know that I have to move ahead and do those things alone that we had planned to do together.'

A few months later Mary wrote me an email from Italy, where she was doing a month-long academic-writing residency. She had postponed and then almost cancelled the long-planned and eagerly anticipated trip that they had originally been going to make together, until her husband fractured his hip. She had agonized about leaving him, even though he had accepted he would be well cared for by their son. And at last, after all the postponements, the anxieties and doubts, she arrived and could sit and look out at the sea, hear the waves pounding the cliff, write and think and feel. It was like 'a long draught of cold water, opening up my mental horizons, with the space and time to think; intensely creative space . . .' she writes. 'I feel as if I've regained my own life and mind.'

Yes, she is acutely aware that she regains her life by – briefly – absenting herself from his. She knows that she is someone who has held on to not being paired, part of a duo: she has travelled on her own, done her own things, 'reserved (not preserved, reserved)' aspects of her own life. 'Maybe it's a lifesaver, but it's also been a problem.' Because the carer of someone with dementia lives between two grave dangers: of withdrawing in order to protect the self, and of becoming extinguished by the needs of the dependent other.

To have one's own life back, if only for a while; to care and yet to psychically survive. How much should one give? *Everything?* One's whole self? It's always too much; it's never enough.

The second woman prefers to remain anonymous. I had never met her before I went to talk to her about her experience of being the carer for her husband, who has dementia, but I felt that I had – or at least felt that she had spoken to me – because I had read and re-read much of what she had written over a long and rich academic career. I love the way she can open doors on to ideas and thoughts that had seemed inaccessible, make connections between things that had seemed unconnected but which under her guidance spring into new life; the way she can think feelingly. Also, she is – like Mary Jacobus – a woman who has thought much about the passing of time, about death, about what it is to be a woman, with a woman's voice, and what it is to be silenced.

She and her husband live in a lovely house with a large garden where spring is just beginning to show, buds pushing through and colour returning. She is in her early eighties now, though age has not dimmed her clarity. We sit in the kitchen, the heart of the house, where there are objects everywhere: books and papers and games and high chairs (she has grandchildren) and mugs and flowers; paintings on the walls: a pile-up of domestic pleasures, of things you look at, read, use. Before we talk and after, I meet her husband, who is thin, a bit stooped, with a lined and nervous face, a kind smile and a courteous manner. He shakes my hand, welcomes me. In his time, he too has been a distinguished academic and writer: he has lived for most of his life in his head. They have been married for over fifty years and have three children. It feels obvious to me, sitting in this place of hospitality and warmth, that they have built up a good life together.

At the beginning of 2016 he had a planned operation for an aneurism that was worrying him. Now of course, with the curse of hindsight, she wishes he had not had it. He was old, he had slowed down somewhat, but he was still functioning and he had just started writing a new book. Later, one of the psychiatrists they saw asked if perhaps there had been a brief stoppage of blood to the brain during the operation. 'Well,' she says, 'I've no will to enquire.'

Whatever the reason, the onset of his dementia was sudden. When he first came home he was more or less all right but quite quickly became very confused and his speech was slurred. After that he was in and out of hospital with urinary infections, and he contracted C. difficile, an infection most often spread in hospital whose symptoms include diarrhoea and nausea. 'By March he was in a really bad way, both physically and cognitively. His speech was so incoherent I rang the doctors and got an emergency assessment: they discovered his kidneys were shutting down. He was put on a drip and returned to a reasonable state. But he was enfeebled. At the beginning of this decline, he would sometimes ask: "What is our future?" and "What is going to become of us?" There was one particular day when he showed that he foresaw his future. Now, he can't read. He can't write. He can't follow a narrative. He can't watch DVDs. He can't go to the cinema. He's so hampered.'

When she looks back she can see that there were signs of cognitive impairment two or three years before he had his operation. He no longer enjoyed going to the cinema because he could no longer 'follow the syntax' of a film. When he had his diagnosis, in March 2016, his previous difficulties were disclosed. 'I think he perhaps compensated for them to a degree nobody had understood. Or why had it come so very quickly?' She grimaces. 'And his tax affairs. Aaaargh!'

She talks with a tender respect of her husband, kindly and with sadness. She is looking back over a long life together, talking always of what used to be. 'He was always very calm and quite silent. You'd have to get through that to know him. If he knew himself what was happening in those years, he didn't indicate it. He was conscious, however, that his long career was in a slow downward arc.'

When he was diagnosed, first in hospital and then at home, he seemed to take no notice at all. She doesn't use the word 'dementia' very much (their Dancing with Dementia class is just their dancing class), and she talks to him of 'an illness you've got that makes it difficult to see how things hang together'. He is no longer continent but seems unperturbed by that – 'he has dissociated. He has coped with shame by making these dissociations and, actually, it's rather successful for him. If I get frustrated he says: "I don't know what you're talking about." He's blocked that whole side off.'

This dissociation goes very deep. 'He has always been very good at it. He has lived so much in his mind. He has been a very devoted writer. All his life, he wrote almost every day. Now he never goes to his writing shed. He doesn't even look at it. I don't think it's conscious, but when he is in the garden he does not glance to the left as he passes it. He has lost that part of his life and he never talks of it. Never.'

A carer comes in the morning to shower and dress him, and again in the evening to wash and undress him. All the rest is her. 'A friend reads to him, but he drifts off to sleep. Music is the thing – he listens to CDs all day long: Schubert, Beethoven quartets, Bach. Mostly chamber music. As soon as one ends he goes on to the next. The grandchildren are a gift: the two-year-old can get through to him: that immediacy is still there. He is polite; he still has a social presence. He still talks a bit, although he has to be prompted all the time. He still laughs. But sometimes he must think he's lost. He is baffled, and he says, "I don't know what's going on. I don't know what this is all about." And once the carer said to him, "Are you OK?" and he said, "No." '

All this time, sitting in her kitchen with mugs of coffee and outside the day brightening in the garden, she has talked of him and never of herself: the wife of over fifty years who has become the carer. I ask her how she manages.

'I'm not sleeping much,' she says mildly. 'He has this habit of poking me. We still sleep in the same bed; we always have done. The most difficult thing is not feeling any physical pleasure, any easy closeness, always having to work at it – because I have other functions now. I'm cleaning him, cooking for us, making arrangements. We were always equal partners.' (I think how painful the past tense is: something irrecoverably gone.) 'Domestic life was very important to us. And we always had a reciprocal relationship. Once, we travelled the world together, visiting other universities, sometimes as the principal and sometimes as the spouse. There was equality. I think of all the things we will never do together again: the theatres, the concerts, the holidays.'

Like Mary Jacobus, she is conscious of needing to hold on to the things in her old life that are precious to her. Although she turns down invitations all the time, she does try to do the things that matter most. (She has just done a 'radical thing' and booked two tickets to the opera.) But she doubts if she will ever write a book again.

Her daughter-in-law said to her recently: 'What if it had been the other way round?' 'If it had been the other way round, I would have gone into a home. It wouldn't have been feasible for him to do for me what I'm doing for him. I think about that.'

Now she knows that the time might be coming when she will no longer be able to continue as his sole carer and her husband will have to go into a home. 'People say he might enjoy it, and the two of us might be able to enjoy time together, if it wasn't twenty-four hours a day.' She tells me of a recent episode when her husband had a terrible seizure. She thought that he was dying. The ambulance arrived, blue lights flashing, and took him to hospital. He was there for a week and 'I had the experience of "another life"', which was in fact like the life she used to possess. 'I got up when I wanted. There were no carers in the house. I thought: "God, there is all that world out there still." I went to two lectures, to a concert. It was like Mephistopheles saying, "All the world is yours." You only have to reach out and grasp it. And then I have a moral reaction: should I?' There is always guilt.

I ask her if she feels she has lost him and she pauses and considers. 'I'm losing him in the sense that I'm turning into someone closer to his mother – and he didn't get on particularly well with his mother! He was always trying to escape her. I am chivvying him. I'm getting him to do things he doesn't want to do. My own mother also had dementia at the end of her life. I was deeply affected when friends of hers said that the real woman had vanished. I thought, "No! She is still my mother. She is still that person." Most of her memory had evaporated or become skewed and partial, and in a sense they were giving themselves permission to sign off on her. But it wasn't true. She was still there. Somewhere.'

Her husband is still there and will always be still there. Somewhere. 'The personhood of a person persists past coherence and past logic. It is in our *frame*; inside of ourselves.'

We have to be able to bear sorrow – not to turn away from it, nor to absorb it or enter into it, but to bear it. Sorrow is a heavy weight.

'I've come past despair,' says Pat Utermohlen's good friend Disie Johnson, who is the sole carer for her husband. 'I have been absolutely despairing. I tried and I tried to keep the person he once was. Now I don't. I've accepted the new one. I'm at a plateau of acceptance, although recently I've started not to enjoy his company. In a way, acceptance is a defeat. I guess the disease has won.' Her husband is, however, 'very happy. I suppose I'm one of the lucky ones. He's in a state of bliss! I seem to be keeping him in ecstasy.' Disie feels 'completely surrounded' by the illness: her 'almost-mother' is in a home with advanced dementia. Her brother and 'greatest pal' has early-onset dementia: not yet seventy, he lies in bed, immobile, his eyes closed, alive and not alive. She talks about her feelings with candour and spirit. She wants to behave properly and she also wants to survive.

For both her and her husband, it was their second marriage, 'unbelievably happy and successful' after their 'disastrous' first ones. He was an economist, an ecologist, a talented amateur painter; handsome, great fun, clever, extroverted, full of conversation and energy. 'We married as soon as we met, we adored each other and we were –' She hesitates, not wanting to sound vain. 'I guess we were a bit of a golden couple for a while.' He was diagnosed when he was seventy-three, when they were living in Italy. Their world – all their plans for the future – was ruptured. 'If he had known what was to become of him he would have –' She slices her hand across her throat. 'Early on he would sometimes say, "Something is wrong; something is terribly, terribly wrong." But now he has absolutely no perception of the seriousness of the situation. He has no connection whatsoever to his dementia. If he sees a programme on television about it, he'll say, "Oh, the poor things." People come in and look after him occasionally, but he has no idea why. He gets a bit worried that I'm having to make all these decisions: "Darling, what can I do to help you?" he'll say. Or, "Darling, do let me carry that case." Or: "Darling, can I come too?" He's always been quite dependent on me – I think women have spoilt him throughout his life – and now he's *completely* dependent. He says: "You're so good to me; I know it must be a bore . . ." I think he's entirely forgotten the person that he used to be. He loves going to bed: he gets in and he says, "This is *heaven*." He says he wants to live until he is ninety.'

They used to talk all the time, and her husband was a 'man of great richness of language'; now he uses stock phrases or doesn't talk at all. 'There's no chat in our lives any more. That's almost the hardest thing: it's *gone*. There's silence – and thank God for Radio 4. And music.' They have a roof terrace in their tiny London flat that she has filled with flowers, and they can look out at red London buses, at trees just now coming into leaf. He sits there and listens to Monteverdi and she reads him poetry and he feels very contented. He has a state-provided carer for one three-hour session a week and anything extra has to be paid for. 'I go out as much as I can. I have to. *I have to*. Do I shout? Of course I shout! And he just smiles at me lovingly says, "Come and sit with me, my darling." He doesn't like me to be at home and not with him. It's *oppressive*. But we still laugh – about his memory, about the way I shout at him, everything. And I think: "If only this was as funny as you think."'

She glares at me: 'I'm *jealous*,' she says. 'That's the truth of it. I'm jealous of friends, of the ones who go out whenever they want, of all my contemporaries. I am not living a normal life; there's nothing normal about it, except the carapace you put around yourself. None of my friends really accompany us through it. People like us are shut out from ordinary life. And of course you resent it. Heidegger said that boredom is when you sense the passage of time – passing time. How could you want that? What life is that?'

She smiles wryly and drinks some of her wine, adding: 'The problem is that he is so very happy – though he doesn't say that, he says, "I am the happiest of men" – and I, well, I am the most miserable.' She sets down her wine. She has a beautiful, strong face; of course they were a golden couple, the world at their feet. 'Miserable and exhausted and desperate. Disjunction is the name of the game.'

Disie is formidable and she is kind. She has undertaken this hard task and is determined to do it well and see it through. At the same time, she knows her own limits and she mocks herself and her failures, mimicking her politely furious voice when she gets impatient (she never mocks or mimics her husband): ' "Darling, get up . . . Darling, could you get up? Darling, I've brought you tea . . . Darling, you haven't drunk your tea . . . Darling, what about getting up now? . . . Darling, change your pants . . . You need to change your pants . . . They're under the basin . . . Darling, you haven't changed them . . ." An hour and a half later it's still going on and *for God's sake*.' She will not be swallowed up by the role of carer. 'Brain work,' she says. 'That's the thing.' She goes to opera courses, language classes, Pat Utermohlen's art classes; she sees friends. When she is at home she gives herself a set of rituals – cooking something nice for lunch and dinner for them both, making their flat pleasant, reciting poetry to her husband, hearing her own voice echo in the silence she has come to dread. She tries to hold the sorrow and the anger and the fear at bay, but every so often she admits to a sense of isolation and hopelessness. She is scared of her own ability to remain equable, scared of losing him even more, this man who she loved so much; loves. 'Which of course I will.'

'I don't remember if I shouted at Bill.' Says Patricia Utermohlen quietly. There's a small pause. She adds: 'I don't want to remember.'

'It's important to talk of, say, hatred, or of murderous feelings,' says the CEO of the Tavistock Centre for Couples Relationships, Andrew Balfour, much of whose work involves supporting couples through the illness that affects one of them and ensuring that they do not feel entirely alone and unsupported. 'If people can't acknowledge that, they may enact it or withdraw and cut off from the relationship. People need their strategies and defences.' He talks of 'containment' theory, usually applied to infants: the idea is that development takes places within a series of relationships. He is careful not to imply that people with dementia are like children, and he dislikes the 'saccharine infantilization' of frail older people, but he says that, like children, they need a kind of containment. 'And the container of someone with dementia needs containment themselves – it's the Russian-doll model. Carers need support if they are to remain emotionally available. If, for instance, you're screamed at over and over again, you need help to tolerate how that makes you feel.' You can't, he believes, do it alone. And it is vital that the carer's work of looking after a person and 'rescuing something meaningful' is properly recognized: too often, he says, it is 'invisible, unremarked, unrecorded'.

Every story is different. I give a talk at Suffolk Family Carers and meet a man who looks after his daughter, who has mental-health problems, and his wife, who has dementia. He cares for them and does the household chores from the moment he gets up to the moment he sleeps. He had to give up work to do this profoundly important job that most people don't recognize as a job; their income has plummeted. He has lost most of his friends and, if he stops to think about it, understands that he is lonely and sad. He is very matter-of-fact. He is just doing his duty. He doesn't understand he is a hero.

I meet a woman whose husband lashes out at her. She knows it is his disease, not him. He was a gentle person before he became ill and perhaps he still is.

I meet a woman who looks after her daughter, who has epileptic fits that are gradually obliterating her, while at the same time looking after her mother with dementia. This woman wears a bright pink knitted hat and a pink scarf and has the kind of wilful, gallant cheerfulness about her that I've seen in other carers.

I meet men and women who are old and not strong but who every day lift their partner, take their weight: it's physical, strenuous work.

I meet children who have taken their parent with dementia into their home and whose lives have been turned upside down.

Children who are caring for a parent who never properly cared for them, even who abused them, when they were young, and it is as if they were in some way restoring order and decency to their world.

Grandchildren who are part-time carers and worrying about how to do well at school as well.

Carers who barely go out themselves any more: home has become a prison; they are waiting out the sentence together.

Carers who have moments of hatred for the person they are caring for, and who hate themselves for hating.

Carers (and this is almost every carer I meet) who feel guilty because they get impatient and lose their temper, or because they sometimes accept help from outside, or because they occasionally go out alone and do things that are just for them, brief moments of selfishness. Selfishness has a bad name – but it can be another word for sanity.

I meet carers who are humorous, optimistic, tender and unresentful, who regard their task as a difficult privilege, something given to them, but who have nevertheless become depressed, ill, angry, poor, chaotic, flattened, trapped, heart-broken, utterly undone and at the end of their tether; they feel that they can't go on and still they go on. And on and on and on. There are hundreds of thousands of them, not saints but ordinary people who too often struggle on alone.

The most unsettling interview that I did turned out to be the one with Tommy and Joyce Dunne, in their neat, cheerful bungalow. It started out as a story of hope in the face of catas-trophe: a man who came through terror and despair and who is now leading a good, purposeful life, trying to make lives better for others who live with the illness; a woman who has been unswervingly loyal and supportive through their mar-riage's terrible ordeal, giving up her work to help him with his; a story of fidelity, courage, resilience and optimism. And it is that story still, but underneath it lies another one, much more complicated.

I had been with them for some time, and for the most part we had talked about Tommy's experience, Joyce helping him in the telling. And perhaps that sense of once more being on the sidelines of his story, not at the centre of her own, was the trigger for what came next. They were describing the play about dementia that Tommy had co-written and that they were both taking part in, and it sounded very jolly. They were smiling, laughing, joking, and out of the blue, quite matter-of-factly, Joyce says: 'I would say we don't have a relationship as a man and wife any longer.'

I stare at her, taken aback.

'No,' she continues. 'Tommy doesn't look at me. And I live on eggshells. He will shout at me about anything.'

She is still smiling. Tommy is also smiling, seemingly unperturbed by her words. I suddenly realize that, all this time they have been sitting together on the sofa, they haven't looked at each other, touched each other, talked to each other. Everything has been directed towards me. Looking back at the transcript of our talk, I examine the pronouns they used (pronouns often give us away: along with prepositions, articles and conjunctions, they are the connective tissue of language and can reveal much more than 'content' words because we use them so often and so unthinkingly.) Tommy never says 'you' to his wife; he doesn't say 'we' or 'us'. He says 'I' and 'she'.

Joyce's words turn a dial in my mind: the performance that had been played out in front of me takes on a different meaning: no longer a movie by Richard Curtis but a play by Pinter or Beckett, a scene about hard, grim loneliness.

'It's true,' Tommy says calmly. 'I can't do reality any more.' He sounds like he's talking about a stranger, one he has no responsibility for.

'And it's sad,' says Joyce. 'It's very, very sad.'

'It's as if all emotions have been stripped away,' Tommy continues, as if she hasn't spoken. 'I can't understand why she needs to be told why she looks nice. It makes no sense. I see it logically but the empathy part doesn't exist. It's been taken away.'

I remember Professor Martin Rossor, clinical neurologist and National Director for Dementia Research, in his pleasant room in Queen Square, telling me about people with dementia who lose empathy and who no longer feel a sense of distress, for others or even themselves. I also remember his saying that perhaps the loss of empathy is what denotes a loss of self. I don't speak: what can I say?

'If I said, "I love you," I'd only be saying it because I'd been told to.' Tommy still isn't looking at Joyce. 'I used to think that she was the sun rising every morning and going down in the evening. I remember that I did feel that once . . . To get home from work and to see her.'

Joyce nods. 'He's no longer interested in me. He never says: *How was your day? Who did you meet? Do you want tea?* It's not worth saying anything to him: sometimes I just go out of the room, count to ten, and then return.'

'But when she goes out' – still not saying 'you' to Joyce, who is talking of heartbreak – 'it's as if she's been out for minutes, not hours. I have no sense of time passing.'

I say something inadequate, about how profound this loss is, a sucker punch the illness had delivered.

'I grieve every day for the person I was,' says Tommy. 'I miss the Tommy I used to be. Sometimes I wake up and I don't recognize Joyce. It frightens me. Like seeing myself in the mirror and thinking it's my father.'

'He gives out the wrong message,' says Joyce. 'He's the most loving person to everyone else. He'll give anyone a hug, tell them they look nice.'

It's true: when they collected me from the station, Tommy hugged me and we linked arms. He felt adorable.

'Well, we always push the closest one away.' Tommy gives this bland assessment smilingly, agreeing with all that Joyce says.

'He's in this Twitter group,' says Joyce. 'He's a different person then! He loves it. I'm looking at him, and he's so excited and like this.' And she makes an animated face and lifts up her hands expressively.

I ask Joyce if she's angry.

'Angry? Oh yes! I know it's the illness, but I'm angry. I can't show it, though: Tommy would just throw something at me.' Tommy nods mildly. 'I love Tommy, but I'm not in love with him any more. He's pushed me further and further away from him.'

Not long ago, she persuaded him to go to marriage counselling with her, but he hated it: 'It was hearing about reality. It was hearing about my failings. There's a difference between knowing how to do something and doing it. I could read a book on how to fly a plane, but I couldn't fly it.'

Their two children are a great support to her: her daughter tells her she must live her own life; her son advises her not to let Tommy control her. 'Because he does. It's because he's losing so much.'

'When she's not there, I miss her,' says Tommy.

'I feel like I'm mourning,' says Joyce.

'It's the long goodbye.'

'But I can't get depressed. I can't. I just get on with it.'

'I cry,' says Tommy.

'I've never once seen you cry!'

'I do, though. When I'm alone. When she's here, I feel safe.'

'I miss so much. Work. The things I used to do and love to do. All our plans. I miss intimacy: a kiss, a cuddle. If I ever try to cuddle him, he'll just give me his cheek, trying to get it over with. But he can't cope if I cry. Never could. I have to push things down and down and down. Sometimes I think he would never stand up for me. It's really hard. It's a terrible,

terrible thing, how it's made us question our whole relationship, which has always been so strong and good.'

'I'm on an escalator. It's quite a slow movement, but it's down.'

'I don't think we've got hopes left,' says Joyce, tearless and bleak.

'Dementia takes hope away.'

'But I'm proud of myself,' says Joyce, '*Very*. No one else would put up with Tommy and, if it was the other way round, Tommy wouldn't be here.'

'I wouldn't. If she'd done to me what I've done to her, I'd have ripped my hair out long ago.'

'I've gone through hell,' says Joyce.

Tommy looks at me sympathetically. 'I know. If you make a film, you want a happy ending, don't you?'

I went away feeling shaken by this interview and by the cruelty of an illness that can attack the very things that are most precious – taking away not only memories and capacities but love. At the start of our meeting Tommy had shown me concentric circles, with the world at the edge, and *I* at the centre. It was as if for Tommy, only *I* remained intact, the links connecting it to humanity fraying and broken. How lonely for him, how lonely for her.

(And this isn't quite a happy ending, but the following day Tommy sent me an email:

> I really enjoyed our talk, but the most important thing I will take away from that is I am not letting dementia beat me, so why should I let it take away my love for Joyce? I am really going to make the effort to get back to the love that

we had, or should I say have, because if you fan a fire that's nearly out you can get it to roar again, so hold the last lines in that chapter.

And several months later he wrote to me again:

It's been hard work every day trying to control the beast that is dementia, but Joyce has been fantastic. She has somehow learned to adjust . . . and accepts that on bad days it's the dementia not Tommy that's speaking and doing things, and has learned that by going with the flow rather than arguing or confronting me she can calm me down. She now understands that none of those things are directed at or meant to hurt her. We now have lots of laughs and plenty of cuddles, therefore we are in a much happier place than we were before we met you and realized that if we didn't make the effort, then something beautiful would be lost.

Joyce wrote to me as well, reiterating what Tommy said:

While it is still hard to see Tommy not be able to do all the things he once did, we are at a happier place at the present moment. I still miss the old Tommy and wish with all my heart that I could have him back, but I know that cannot be. We try to enjoy all the time we have together and I enjoy going to the various groups with him, as I know that to really enjoy quality time with him I've got to enter into his world. There are a few bad days when dementia wins, but the good days help make up for them. The most important thing is to never give up. I wake up every day and hope that Tommy is still here and that he knows me.

In this stoic message, a phrase stands out: 'I've got to enter into his world.' There's the carer's perpetual dilemma: how much to hold on to the old world, the independent self, and how much to relinquish that in order to be kind, to be loyal, to keep a relationship alive, to care.

'Hold the last lines in that chapter,' Tommy had written in his previous email. Full of admiration and disquiet, fearful with hope, I'm holding.)

8. *Connecting through the Arts*

'And hand in hand, on the edge of the sand,
They danced by the light of the moon.'

My father loved to dance; as a young man, he'd been a nimble,
fluent dancer and, old, his body still remembered all the steps
and he was light on his feet. At Sean's fiftieth-birthday party in
Sweden, my father took to the floor and blithely danced the
tango, proud of his agility, steering his surprised partners
around the old barn. He loved to sing and from time to time
he would sit at the piano we had for a few years and pick out
tunes, jazzy, ragtime, improvised, the tip of his tongue on his
lip in happy concentration. He liked painting, usually land-
scapes and still lifes in watercolour, but occasionally swift
sketches in charcoal. Even during his last holiday in Sweden
with us, he would sit with a paint palette and spiral-bound
pad, looking out at the lake and the trees, occasionally dipping
his brush in bright colour and trailing it across the thick paper.
And he took pleasure in reading stories and poetry aloud, acting things out, boyish in his unself-conscious enthusiasm. In
some ways, he was a shy man, but there was a buoyancy and
confidence about his everyday creativity – as if the flow of life,
in and out like breath, was unimpeded.

In his last terrible months there would be music playing in
his little room downstairs, and we often read poems to him:
the same ones each time, the ones he had read to us many

years previously. 'The Owl and the Pussycat', Ogden Nash fragments that used to tickle him, 'The Highwayman', 'I Wandered Lonely as a Cloud,' 'If' – all the golden oldies. One time, I went into his room with Sean and all my four children and we read – chanted, really, raggedly in unison – 'I must go down to the seas again, to the lonely sea and the sky' – and he, who could no longer speak, joined in . . . We kept going, leaning towards him, smiling, tears running down our cheeks; he remembered the ends of lines, the words that rhymed, phrases and little fragments of freedom and friendship and death: 'the lonely sea and the sky', 'steer her by', 'all I ask', 'sweet dream when the long trick's over' . . . In that tangled-up, snarled-up, muddled-up mind where everything seemed blocked off, barriers thrown up around the wreckage to prevent exit and entrance, the roar of the world beyond him, the memory of words he had loved long ago still delicately chimed. Moments like this were a gift – to him, and to us as well, miraculous spaces of reciprocity that opened up between us.

I don't know if this was happy or sad. It makes me want to howl. But I do know that art can seem magical in the way that it can find a person who had seemed quite lost. A golden thread weaving its way through the razed civilization, the rubble and chaos and shattered meanings, and a light glimmers in the darkness and a voice speaks. *I am here. I am here. I was always here.*

A few months ago, turning on the radio, I heard a voice saying that creative writing can help wounds heal faster. Startled, I turned the volume up. Volunteers were given small cuts; half were then asked to write about something distressing in their life, the other half about something mundane. The wounds of the confessional writers healed substantially more quickly.

A thought or a feeling is felt on the skin. Our minds, which have power over our bodies, are in our bodies and are our bodies: we cannot separate the two. Words, self-expression, can tangibly help pain and suffering. Art can be medicine, for body and soul.

William Utermohlen, after he was diagnosed with dementia, withdrew in loneliness and terror into his own shrinking world. But the day came when he picked up his brush once more and for the next few years he made, in his astonishing self-portraits, a journal of self-loss that remains unique: the *I* observing the *I* that is disappearing. They are artistic, medical, psychological documents. They show the battle to preserve his identity as an artist and as a human being, uncannily occupying the interior world of the artist and also the exterior world that watches him. William Utermohlen had always expressed himself through his art, and with these self-portraits he was in communication with the world once again, and the world was in communication with him.

At the Wellcome Foundation, Dr Seb Crutch – a neuro-psychologist who was once one of William Utermohlen's physicians – is heading a project called 'Created out of Mind'. He wants to both 'enrich our perceptions' of what it is to live with dementia, presenting it instead as a multiplicity of diverse and not always or inevitably distressing symptoms, and also to explore the ways in which art can enrich the lives of people who live with the illness. Not art as a hobby, or a way of passing the time, but art as a way of unleashing everyday creativity and helping people remain part of the world's intricate web of communication.

In the Wellcome Foundation's airy Hub, high above the roar of London's traffic-clogged Euston Road, Seb Crutch talks with animation about how we should learn to value the experience of people living with the illness: 'We want to be *inspired* by people with dementia,' he says. 'There might be scariness, sadness, depression, but there is also intrigue, interest, uncertainty. Our bias is towards the idea that there is value in the experience.'

People sometimes think, he says, that 'the arts should make us happy. No! Music, for instance, can confirm the mood we're in; confirm our sadness. It is allowing us to plug in to our inner selves.' And he adds, 'The arts should be done *with*, not *to*.' It's about collaboration, engagement, embodied knowledge, everyday creativity, the porous boundaries between the self and other, living in the moment. Music, words, pictures have the power to take you to a different place, like a kind of magic carpet.

When I talk to Alex Coulter of South-West Arts, who was a member of an all-party Parliamentary group looking into the benefits of the arts upon health and well-being, she reiterates this power of the arts to take us both into our self and into the world. After two years of evidence gathering, roundtables and discussions with service users, health and social care professionals, artists and arts organizations, academics, policy makers and parliamentarians from all parties and both houses, its unambiguous findings are that the arts can help keep us well, aid our recovery and support longer lives better lived; they can help us meet major challenges facing health and social care – ageing, long-term conditions, loneliness and mental health; and they can help save money in the health service and in social care. She tells me of an experience that the violinist Neil Valentine had: a woman in a hospital side-room was so disturbed that the staff could do nothing for her. He played his violin very quietly, over and over again, and gradually she was quietened and comforted. Something was happening: she was enabled to find a calm place inside herself.

It makes sense that one of the major risk factors for dementia is loss of hearing, because this cuts a person off from their world. They retreat into themselves. As Alex Coulter says, 'What we need most of all is connection.'

Many of the people I have spoken to in the course of researching and writing this book – those with dementia and those who care for them – set against the desolation, fear, frustration and muddle this healing and transformative power of art. They talk of it in almost religious terms: of being 'saved' by music, like a gush of clear water in the desert. For as long as was possible, William Utermohlen painted, making shapes and meanings to keep the shapeless and the meaningless at bay. Emptiness and terror were knocking at the door, but still he painted. Disie Johnson's husband listens to music and she reads poetry to him. Jenni Dutton's mother was collaborator, muse and consultant for her daughter's haunting 'Dementia Darnings'. Theresa Clarke writes poetry, though rarely now. Rebecca Myer's father danced with her mother, taking her in his arms and returning them both to their courting days. We live in our bodies and our bodies remember; they respond.

In Sheffield I go to a dance class for people with dementia, where the teacher hands out ribbons, each end held by people at opposite sides of the circle. While we twirl and stomp around the space, we weave our coloured strips, gathering people together, making patterns, linking strangers – a visible reminder of what we are trying to do, which is to connect.

And a few weeks later, in a large hall in London, I hold hands with a tiny woman from Jamaica and a large man from Birmingham, and once more we dance. Bit by bit, our self-consciousness falls away and we grin at each other, laugh. Dementia has robbed them of their verbal ability – but there are many different languages, many different forms of embodied knowledge and ways that we can communicate with each other. The tiny woman is a beautiful dancer; music flows through her. She must have danced throughout her life. I try to imitate her, to borrow some of her lightness and grace. She's showing me, being my teacher; her feet make tricksy movements on the wooden boards. For a while, we are all occupying the same space in the world, so that our categories dissolve. The carer isn't the carer any more; the person with dementia isn't someone who is hampered by incapacity; I'm not the observer. We're equal, active and reciprocal and the music that is flowing through us unites us.

Or, sitting in a church in Essex on a Sunday in June, I look across at my friend Julia's mother. She is in her nineties and has dementia. There are days when she is wretched, chaotic and scared, but each Sunday she is soothed and even enraptured by the experience of singing the hymns that she sang when she was a girl. The music has worn grooves in her memory and, while she may not be able to speak in full sentences any more, she can sing 'Abide with Me' in a true voice and her face, lifted up, looks young, eager, washed clean of anxiety. Julia thinks that at these moments her mother's brain comes together, 'like a flower reviving when it's being soaked in water.' People with dementia, she says, need to be drenched in art.

A friend sends me a YouTube film about the 'Song-a-minute Man'. He has dementia; he can't remember very much any more – but, oh wow, he can remember the songs he has been singing all his life. He and his son are in a car, and they belt out the words. He has a rich, true, full-throttle voice and a smile that would light up a room. The two of them are exuberant, grinning and singing and trying to outdo each other, caught up in the moment. Dementia is nowhere to be seen. (As Tommy

Dunne says: 'I may have dementia but I'm not going to let dementia have me.')

It's what is happening with the chamber orchestra Manchester Camerata's 'Music in Mind', or with 'Music for a While', a project led by Arts and Health South West with the Bournemouth Symphony Orchestra, with Wigmore Hall's participatory 'Music for Life', with the project 'A Choir in Every Home' and 'Singing for the Brain'; with dance classes in hospitals and residential homes; with art galleries and museums that encourage those with dementia to come and talk about art.

I attend one of the monthly sessions at the Royal Academy, modelled on New York's Museum of Modern Art's 'Meet me at MOMA' project led by two practising artists, where people with dementia who have been art lovers through their life and are art lovers still come to talk about a particular work. We sit in front of an enigmatic painting that we are told at the end of the session is by John Singer Sargent, and there is an air of calmness, patience and, above all, time. There are no wrong opinions here, for there are many ways of seeing. People with dementia are continually contradicted and corrected, but in this humanizing democratic space people are encouraged to see, think, feel, remember and express themselves. Slowly at first, they begin to talk. They describe the painting – three women dressed in white in a formal walled garden, a mysterious statue at the end of the path that the eye is drawn to; outside the walls a dark mass of trees. One man thinks we are looking at a harem; another believes it is a garden somewhere Mediterranean (it turns out he's right: this is Italy). One man stands up and points his trembling stick. 'There,' he says. 'That's where the eye is drawn. Through there.' The stick wavers.

'Good and bad,' says another man. 'At end of death; he himself didn't do as well as he should have done.'

His wife, who is his carer, quietly intervenes: 'He's thinking of the American art critic Bernard Berenson,' she says.

'It might be raining,' someone says, looking at the cloudy mass of trees in the painting, beyond the wall. 'Soon it will rain.'

'It looks like the back end of a horse,' says another, to a ripple of laughter. He grins, pleased with himself.

'The trees isolate the central part of the painting.' The man with the stick points again. 'Those bits outside have no meaning whatsoever. Even the women are quite meaningless.' He seems suddenly angry.

I remember something that Andrew Balfour told me, about a piece of work he did with his patients with dementia. He showed them photographs and asked them to describe what they were looking at. There was a match group of people who were not cognitively impaired. One of the photos was of Yehudi Menuhin as a boy, playing a violin. 'The people with dementia said things like: "He's deaf . . . he's very deaf . . . there are tears in his violin." These people saw damage in the boy and in his instrument. It was very poignant.'

(And yet at the end of the Royal Academy session, one of the artists leading the discussion talks about the 'Sargent void' that critics perceive in his work: so the man with the stick was right after all.)

'The women are all going off in a huff,' adds another member of the group. 'They're saying: We've had enough.'

They are making up little stories and they are searching for clues. They talk about focus and where the line is drawn and I'm learning about how to look.

'There's a line that's cutting you off,' says one, and I see that there is; the eye is halted. 'It's stopping the women from getting to the statue, which is something very precious. There's something in the way.'

Is he talking of the painting in front of us or of himself? Everyone is looking for signs, listening to each other and responding. There is a clear sense of language returning, thoughts feeding off each other. They are heard with respect and are validated.

Validation is crucial. We are social beings and exist in dialogue; we all need to be recognized. In health, in wealth, in happiness, in youth and in vigour, we live in a world rich with meanings that we can call upon as a conductor calls upon the orchestra, and are linked to each other by a delicate network of communications. This is what it is to be human: we need to reach out to each other across all that separates us; communication as ropes thrown across the abyss between self and other. The arts can come to our rescue when traditional language begins to fail: to sing, to dance, to put paint on paper, making a mark that says *I am still here*, to be touched again (rather than simply handled), to hear music or poems that you used to hear when you were a child, to be part of the great flow of life.

I remember Sean's Swedish grandfather, who I only met once, shortly before he died. He had dementia and could barely speak. But he could still play the piano, his fingers moving up and down the keys. Embodied memory; memory at his fingertips; music flowing from him. I remember seeing an old woman half carried into a room where her siblings waited: she looked thin as a bird in winter and close to death, but then her siblings began to sing a song they knew as children, long ago. Like a miracle, she revived; her face softened and became younger, her eyes brightened, and she smiled and then she sang.

The film *Alive Inside* was made about a music project in a huge care home in the US. Family and carers are asked about the music the person with dementia used to love, and then this is played to them. An old man with severely advanced dementia sits slumped in a wheelchair. He drools; his eyes are half closed and it's impossible to know if he is asleep or awake. A few times a day, soft food is pushed into his mouth. We see photos of him when he was young; strong and handsome. He loved Louis Armstrong: his daughter remembers he would dance her to school, swinging around lamp posts and singing. Someone puts earphones on the man's head and suddenly the music from his glory days is pouring into him. His old head lifts. His foggy eyes open and knowledge comes into them. His toothless mouth splits into a beatific grin. And now he is dancing in his chair, swaying. And then this man – who doesn't speak any longer – is actually singing. The music has reached him, found him, gladdened him and brought him back into life.

It's like a miracle – but one that happens every day, in care homes, in community halls, in hospitals, wherever kind and imaginative people are realizing that the everyday creativity is not an add-on to the basic essentials of life but woven into its fabric. Oliver Sacks wrote that 'the function of scientific medicine . . . is to rectify the "It" '. Medical intervention is costly, often short term and in some cases can be like a wrecking-ball swinging through the fragile structures of a life. But art calls upon the *I*. It is an existential medicine that allows a person with dementia to be a subject still.

If it was me, if it will be me, I want Matisse's cut-outs and Bach's violin partitas. I want Lucinda Williams singing 'Are You Alright?' in her gravelly drone, which always makes me cry. Leonard Cohen, Bob Dylan, Mozart. Kate and Anna McGarrigle's 'Heart Like a Wheel' over and over again, and their swimming song. I want music I heard when I was young and music my children heard when they were young and we sang together in the car on long journeys. I want music I danced to long ago, and I want to dance again, like I did when I was young. And I want Sean to read me poems by Louis McNeice and Elizabeth Bishop – 'the art of losing isn't hard to master'. Shakespeare ('Fear no more the heat o' the sun'). Nonsense verse. Words and music to seek me out and find me, wherever I have gone.

9. Home

'You can go home again . . . so long as you understand that home is a place where you have never been.'

Not long after we had met, the writer and academic who chose to remain anonymous finally acknowledged that it was no longer possible for her to look after her husband in their family home.

The descent towards helplessness is uneven and unpredictable: you think you're on a straight road towards a known destination but it turns out to be a narrow path winding its way along a cliff edge, full of pitfalls, zigzags, vertiginous views. There often comes a day when something that was being managed becomes unmanaged and unmanageable. Routines are no longer sufficient; days lose their safe shape and turn unruly and full of ugly surprises. The person with dementia may become more confused or distressed, angrier or more agitated. Their body betrays them and their memory lets them down. They need more care than a carer can possibly give – and when the carer gives that as well, they need still more, and so it goes.

But the decision that the time has come for them to move into a home is almost always profoundly painful, often couched in terms of hard necessity and bitter defeat. *I had to . . . There was no choice . . .* Even when it is clearly the right call, the only one, for everyone, the sense of failure is often very marked in these conversations – which are conversations about loss. Something ends: married life, self-possession, being part of the thick flow of the world. We leave home when we are young, starting our own life, making a new home for ourselves. And then we may leave home when we are old – but now it's about the closing of something, a goodbye. However positive the change turns out to be, it marks the ending of a stage of life. The threshold is crossed; the door shuts. That was once home.

We take home for granted until we don't have one. It's not just an address, a roof, bricks and mortar, comfort, a key to a door, a place to lay your head and cook your meals and welcome your friends. Home is existential: a deep human impulse and an anchoring sense of belonging and of being. Just as some biologists think that a bird's nest can be interpreted as an extension of the bird's brain, which happens to make use of bits and pieces of the outside world rather than electrical impulses, so the self continues beyond the barriers of the body. To make a home is a way of continuing the self into the outside world and at the same time of gathering the world safely in and wrapping it around the raw and naked self like a blanket.

My first marriage ended when my two eldest children were just two and not yet one, and so they spent their whole remembered childhood moving between different houses, with their teddy bear and panda accompanying them. Both houses were their unequivocal homes and yet I knew at the time, and they told me much later when they had come through the worst of it, that for many years they were homesick wherever they were, always filled with longing. Whenever we went away, staying in a rented house or a hotel, my daughter would methodically unpack her things into the drawers and arrange books on shelves, even if we were staying only for one night (in this way, lots of things got left behind on our journeys). Sometimes on walks she would insist on collecting up all the sticks she came across to take back to her room (in this way, in the Swedish forests of our summers, walks became slow and fraught affairs). She needed to make a home wherever she might be, using as props the comfort of things. She does it still; I do it as well. Cleaning, planting, filling the fridge, laying a place at the table, lighting candles, pulling down the blinds: it's not (only) a domestic chore but a way of feeling secure in my world, arranging stuff around me so that I've made my own nest.

Almost two decades ago, while I was working on a piece for the *Observer* newspaper, I stayed a day and a night in a care home for people who were old and in many cases had dementia. It was a clean, well-run place; the people who lived there were looked after with kindness and imagination. I couldn't fault it. But lying in my narrow bed that night, I felt a pang of desolation at the thought that this was how my own life might end one day: in a home, but far from home.

Gerard de Vries has a set of criteria that will indicate if the time has come for him to die. One of these, which he mentions to me several times, is the need to go into a home. The care home in which his mother-in-law lives is impeccable: when I visit it with Pauline, it feels more like a boutique hotel. It is an old building in the historic centre of the city, with a park on its doorstep, a dining room which is also open to the public, light flooding in through the large windows, a feeling of airy cleanliness and order. No stench of urine here, no one wandering untended and distressed down dingy corridors. It is well staffed; there are numerous activities. All the residents

(I'm slipping into the jargon – you're not a resident *at* home, only *in* a home) are dressed in nice clothes, hair carefully done. There are flowers everywhere, paintings. This is not a private home but a publicly funded one. Those with pensions pay a part of their monthly income; those without are covered by social security, so it is open to anyone who lives with a certain level of dementia.

I sit at a table in one of the living rooms next to Pauline's mother. She smells nice, of the perfume that Pauline gives her and makes sure she puts on. A woman walks past pushing a little buggy with a baby doll in it. Nearby, a man who was once a famous musician sits slumped on the chair: CDs of his music are on the shelves. Pauline's mother fiddles with the buttons on her blue lacey top and smiles, but smiles at nothing; Pauline holds her hand and smiles as well. When we leave she is visibly moved. 'I feel guilty for my mother's state,' she says. 'She is not dignified. She has lost everything she was. She is in this beautiful home. But every time I leave her I leave her alone. I feel guilty: I have left her there, knowing that she had wanted to prevent living this way. She is helpless in every way and I am guilty all the time. And in some ways, it isn't good that she is round the corner, because she's too near to me to distance myself from this feeling, which is overwhelming. And of course,' she adds, always scrupulously honest, 'it will be a relief to one day not have this feeling that I am leaving her there, in this beautiful place, in this awful situation.'

What a difference a letter makes. 'Home' is a small word meaning the centre of one's world, the place from which one sets out that is 'at the heart of the real'. 'A home' in many cases doesn't mean safety at all but removal and unbelonging. Home is domestic and personal; a home, however welcoming and homely, is professional and institutional. Home is where you are in control of your life; a home is where your life is partially or wholly arranged for you, and maybe not in the way that you desire. Home is where you live, and a home is usually the place you go before you die. For some it is the last refuge; for others a waiting room where you don't want to be but don't want to leave. One by one, you're summoned.

'Show me the way to go home, I'm tired and I want to go to bed.' We are in a residential care home for people with dementia in Oxfordshire, seated in a circle, singing. A young woman with a guitar and a glorious fall of red hair leads us. The woman next to me is lusty, her voice clear, her swollen hands tapping out the rhythm; the man opposite in his wheelchair looks slightly dazed but he mouths the words. Most of us are singing, though some sit silently. I look from face to face and wonder what they are thinking, what they are feeling. 'Wherever I may roam, on land or sea or foam,' we sing. The woman next to me reaches out and pats me on the arm, as if to comfort me. '. . . You can always hear me singing this song: show me the way to go home.'

Where is home for them? Are they at home here, now? Or is home somewhere else, in the past and forever gone? Where is home for Eddy Bell's mother, who thinks she is running the one she is in and has sherry in the bath and other people's dolls locked up in her wardrobe? Where is home for the woman in the hospital bed who pleads, over and over again, to be taken there? Or for the woman who runs away from her care home, wanting to get there? Where was it for my father, when he lay in his hospital bed downstairs, the bird table outside his window, and told us it was time to go there? Home is where they speak your language: by language, I do not mean just words but that which connects the inner self with the outer world. When all language falls away, nowhere is familiar.

The building of a house and the idea of dwelling on the earth are intimately connected (*bauen*, to build, and 'being' have the same roots). Without a home, one is 'shelterless' and lost in 'non-being'. Emigration means not only crossing the water and living among strangers but 'undoing the very meaning of the world and – at its most extreme – abandoning oneself to the unreal, which is also the absurd'.

In his film *Human Flow*, the Chinese artist Ai Weiwei follows the movements of the 65 million people who have no home. It's a vision of populations in flight, trekking down mountain roads and across deserts, crammed into open boats to cross the Mediterranean, sleeping in ditches, under bridges, in tent cities, pressed up against tall wire fences, a staggering mass migration of people who are searching for a home, and all they have is what they can carry. They are on a quest; they urgently need their journey to have an end. As that much-missed philosopher of hospitality John Berger once wrote, home is not primarily a dwelling but an emotion and an identity, the 'untold story of a life being lived'. It is preserved through habits – jokes, opinions, actions, gestures, 'the raw material of repetitions turned into a shelter', while memory is the 'mortar that binds the improvised home together'. Within it, tangible mementoes are arranged. 'Home becomes the 'return to where distance did not yet count'. And Hisham Matar, in his moving memoir of his dead father, experiences his return to his childhood home in a similarly self-centring way, as 'a precise and uncomplicated conviction the world was available to me. But wasn't this an odd thing to think, now that I was finally home? Or is this what being home is

like: home as a place from which the entire world is suddenly
possible?'

What makes a home into *home*? What makes a resident into a
member of a new family and an institution into a place of welcome and belonging? Over the past few years I have visited a
great many residential homes, at home and abroad, and each
time I step over the threshold I feel an anticipatory lowering of
the spirits, a kind of muted dejection. Large, medium and
small; modern builds and converted old ones. Long corridors.
Careful lighting. Matching, wipeable furniture, frequently in
beige or in red. Hoists and stair lifts. Photos of younger selves
on the walls. Photos of flowers, blown up large, and of tranquil
water. Sometimes there's a smell of urine, or worse; mostly
these places are clean. I have been to music sessions, dancing
classes, I've done the hokey-cokey and twisted again, like we
did last summer. I've talked with the people who live there,
who work there, sat in dining rooms and sitting rooms and
bedrooms. The staff in these places are usually low paid, often
on the minimum wage or zero-hours contracts, and their crucial work is barely recognized. Many of them show great
kindness and patience towards their vulnerable residents,
going beyond mere duty, and some of them seem genuinely to
be enjoying their job and taking pleasure in the company of
those they are caring for.

But I've only been to the homes that wanted me to visit
them and were prepared for me – available for inspection.
'Home' might be a word for safety and belonging; it is also
where most of life's bad stuff happens. Cruelty and violence
don't usually take place out in the streets, done by strangers,
but in those private, hidden spaces where we can't observe it
or prevent it, behind closed doors, and against people who are

powerless. Abuse flourishes in intimate, secret places, close to home.

In the US, there are apparently more than 2 million cases of elder abuse each year in nursing homes; one in ten old people will experience some form of abuse. People with dementia are much more likely to be abused than those without it. What's more, elder abuse is probably the most under-reported form of violence in the country.

It's the same depressing story in the UK, where the care system is under severe pressure, with many experts saying it is disintegrating: home-care workers are paid paltry amounts of money to spend tiny amounts of time in the homes of the old and vulnerable. There have been over 23,000 allegations of home-care abuse in the last three years – which means there must be more, because often the people who are being abused can't tell tales (which, of course, is partly why they are being abused). Many care homes are understaffed and operating within a punitive, impossible budget; the tens of thousands of allegations of abuse over the last three years include neglect, physical abuse, psychological abuse and sexual abuse.

All over the world, in poor countries and rich ones, hundreds and thousands of old and vulnerable people live the last part of their life in fear and distress, in loneliness and in sorrow.

Even where there is no overt mistreatment it isn't uncommon for people to be treated as objects, spoken over and about, not to, and stripped of all autonomy. Although when I've visited residential homes everyone was aware I was there as a writer, journalist and watching eye, I've nevertheless witnessed staff being sluggish and indifferent towards those in their care. They seemed not to notice distress, or dismissed agitation as a person being 'difficult' – like a child behaving badly. I think they have genuinely ceased to notice that these people are depressed or purposeless (indeed, for many people, old age is almost synonymous with depression) or that they are lonely. 'The package of care' is often the package of loneliness. As Atul Gawande writes, 'We end up with institutions that address any number of societal goals . . . but never the goal that matters to the people who reside in them: how to make life worth living when we're weak and frail and can't fend for ourselves any more.' The adult children who often choose the homes prioritize safety. For the people who have to live there, other things might be more important: autonomy, for instance, or sociability, or *fun*. I know about all the health and safety regulations, the necessary bureaucracy of professional care – but why can't everyone who wants and is able cook together, or keep hens in the garden, have dogs and cats and other animals, be in charge of their own life as far as possible, with a purpose to each day? Being kept safe is a tiny part of what makes a home.

Things are changing from the days that my grandmother was in a home, where the dark hall was thick with the ammonia stench of urine overlaid with air freshener, and where residents spent their days sitting around the edges of rooms, half asleep, occasionally being given jolly, time-passing, soul-destroying activities to do (bingo, jigsaws . . .). Increasingly, there are homes that allow pets – and why not? Alcohol with meals – and why not? A coming and going of the residents, because, after all, that's what they've always done. There are homes that are built on the grounds of schools or colleges; homes where young people volunteer, where residents are stakeholders, helping to select staff. Homes where the people who live there are in control of their days as far as possible.

Probably (I don't know), more residential homes are good than not-good. Although a handful are downright appalling, quite a few are outstanding, and in these places of refuge and companionship, people may flourish again.

For twenty weeks in 2013, the poet Sarah Hesketh visited a residential care home for people with dementia as part of an artist-in-residence programme. The men and women who lived at the Lady Elsie Finney House in Preston had advanced dementia; some were dying there. It was, she says, 'a surreal environment'. There were 'weird things on walls' – stickers of portholes with seagulls perched on them; heart-shaped posters; a skeleton wearing a pair of glasses. People were locked into their rooms. Many of the staff, she says, 'were great' and several opened up to her, telling her how hard their job was and how unrecognized. At the end of her first day she felt scared and sad; 'I kept being sad but I never felt scared again.' At the Elsie Finney House, 'Nobody thought they were in the place they lived in.' They found ways to explain why they were there: one woman believed she was back at school and the staff were her teachers. (I think of Jan Bell happily thinking she was running the home where she lives). Sarah Hesketh says that no one went out into the garden in the nine months she was going there, and that there was a sense of living on the far edges of life. Hospitals are often at the centre of things ('choirs and MPs visit them'), but 'homes are on the margins', so there is often a sense of being 'shut away out of sight; of loneliness'. Old age can push people to the edge of society; dementia often pushes them right out of sight, and then out of mind. They are the missing persons.

I visit a newly opened residential home in Berkshire, home to sixty or so women and men with dementia. It is made up of circular buildings and is flooded with light. As soon as I step into its fresh, clean, bright space, flowers everywhere, I am filled with relief. Such care and imagination has gone into its design. Each bedroom has its own numbered front door with a window next to it that holds objects and pictures the resident has chosen and a back door that opens on to a courtyard. There are small living rooms, a cinema, a real shop; there's a well-being room; there are nooks with armchairs in them. There are books on shelves, and interesting objects; pictures and puzzles. It's being home by mimicking home. The circular structure means there are no dead ends: people can walk and walk without getting lost or being brought to a halt. There's a large garden and a gardening club. There's a playground where grandchildren can play, watched over by their grandparents. And I'm struck by how staff hold and embrace and *touch* the old people they are caring for: so often old people are touched only when they are being washed and fed, and then it is often by gloved hands. The people who live there are part of the staff-selection process. At night, staff wear pyjamas so that if someone wakes they will know it is not time to get up. And, crucially, family and friends are welcome there at all times, even for the night. Of course, people still get upset and they still get homesick: sometimes for the place they have recently left, more often existentially – for their childhood, their parents, their old sense of safety and hope, of life unfolding in front of them. 'You try to enter their world,' says the manager. 'You have to pay attention to small things, give them dignity, respect, their autonomy. You have to know each person.'

I meet a man of ninety-nine who still misses his dead wife sorely but who is less lonely now he is in a home. He's making new friends (youngsters in their eighties). I dance with a woman with piercing blue eyes and a smile that never leaves her small face who tells me her life is 'smashing' now she has left her own home, where time passed very slowly. A home is not often home, but care may be care – kindness in action – and in many homes there is great kindness and endeavour. At every stage in life people need to feel they have a purpose and a part to play, and recently I've been struck by the courage and optimism people have in the face of loneliness, frailty and profound loss. A home can become home. Or nearly.

Mary Jacobus tells me how at the workshops she has been to in Ithaca carers are advised 'never to say never'. And Raymond Tallis is adamant that, far from resisting the conditional idea of his elder forgetful self in a home, he welcomes it. 'I *do* want to go to a home. I want to say to Terry [his wife]: "I don't want you to remember me, after forty-seven years together, through a prism of three years of hell. Being a degraded body that's behaving badly."' He chuckles. 'I think maybe she should sign a contract to that effect.'

When we talk of residential homes, there can be a whiff of the poorhouse, of warehousing the powerless. The clues are in the language: we speak of 'sending' people to a home, as if to boarding school or even prison; of 'putting them' there, as if they had become an object; of 'residents'. Their world shrinks: from a house or flat, say, to a room, just a few possessions remaining and everything else left behind, or sold, or handed on; photos on the wall as reminders of what life once was. Then just to a chair by the window. To a bed . . .

For Rebecca Myers and her family, the decision that her mother should go into a home was 'terrible', although they had reached a stage that was unsustainable. They all visited her, and until she died Rebecca's father went every day and never stopped loving her. But 'he met someone', Rebecca says. The woman worked in the home where her mother was. She and her father started a relationship. 'And Mum was still there, still alive.' She looks at me searchingly; there's no anger or resentment in her voice. 'It was *hard*. I could see how lonely he was. And he became happy again – there was always that sorrow there, but he laughed once more. So I'm grateful to the woman.'

It's the reverse situation to the one portrayed in the film *Away from Her*, in which Julie Christie plays a woman with early-onset dementia who goes into a home. Watched by her anguished husband, she becomes romantically involved with another resident. Is it infidelity? Of course it isn't. Of course it is. As Rebecca says, it's *hard*.

Maggie East weeps when she talks about her beloved husband Denis East leaving home. 'I said, "I can't do it." I left him there.'

Denis East was a gifted violinist who played in the BBC Symphony Orchestra, the Boyd Neel Orchestra and the Yehudi Menuhin Bath Festival Orchestra, as well as teaching at the Trinity College of Music. In the fifties he founded the Denis East Quartet, and later he played in a quartet with some of his students, who continued to play as a trio after he went into the home.

He was many years older than Maggie and their affair and marriage caused a family rift. She talks of him with anguish and pride, showing me photographs of her husband as a handsome young man, dark-haired and solemn, his violin in his hands. His life had always been soaked in music. He was something of a prodigy, winning a scholarship at fifteen to study at the Royal College of Music. And music literally saved his life: as a Japanese prisoner of war in his early twenties, he escaped hard labour by playing at concert parties. (She shows me a dog-eared programme for a concert at Changi jail – and there's his name, Denis East paying Chopin, Paganini, Bach.) When he had terrible ulcers, he was scheduled to have his hands amputated until the surgeon discovered he was a violinist and saved them. He was a 'big, tall man' who came home weighing seven stone and carrying an enduring terror of being locked into places – of being a prisoner once again – and who cried every time his friend George Wall with the beautiful voice was mentioned.

Denis East was known to his friends as 'the memory man': he didn't just remember his own part but all the orchestral parts. In the camp, he would copy scores out from memory. And when his own memory began to fail he was angry, scared and frustrated, banging his head against the wall and shouting. (She shows me another photo of her husband, once more with his violin, but now his hair is silver. And another, wearing a red jumper and holding a glass in both hands, as if to steady it; his expression has become one of a familiar strained anxiety.) Maggie was still working as a primary-school teacher and Denis East's minder was George, their Great Dane/Labrador cross ('a medium Dane', says Maggie), who kept his master on track for a while: 'Every morning, Denis would take George for a walk, buy ham from the village shop and put it in the fridge, go upstairs to his studio with George, play his violin until midday, at which point George would lay his head on Denis's bow arm and show him it was time for lunch. Ham for George, sandwich for Denis.'

And then the faithful dog died (just as Theresa Clarke's dog died and left her to her confusion) and things began to unravel. Her husband started to get lost. He would 'walk and walk and walk'. At the memory clinic, where he knew he couldn't get out, he would climb over a high wall (a scared old man) and escape 'like from prison. He wanted to come home.' But home was starting to have a different meaning – not just Maggie and their converted chapel in Suffolk but also his childhood. 'He became obsessed by the need to see his long-dead parents who lived in London: 48 Mora Road. I took him there once and he didn't recognize it. He was always wanting to walk back to London, up on to the A134, going home to his long-ago past – although when he had returned from his terrible war, emaciated, traumatized and stricken, his parents didn't welcome him back. They had been told he was dead, and when he appeared like a ghost his father simply said: "I don't know what your mother's going to say." ' Maggie says he never got over that. Yet still he yearned to return to his childhood self, there in suburban Cricklewood, before the world became a savage, heartbreaking place.

(Claire Kent at the Tavistock Centre talks of how people with dementia will often search for their earliest home – when they're tired, when they're anxious or confused, they want that place of safety. They go out at night especially, looking. Looking for what? Looking for something, but what is it? They've lost something: themselves?')

Denis East was often agitated and could be physically violent. Maggie sometimes locked him in to keep him safe (she falters as she tells me this). One day he escaped and brought the traffic on the A134 to a standstill. 'Denis was weaving about on the road. There were about six people trying to stop him; he was pushing them away; he was trying to push his carer into the oncoming traffic. I persuaded him I would drive him to Mora Road – and then I drove him home. I bolted all the doors and he said: "You realize we're locked in here? Trapped?" We were trapped together. A neighbour came round and asked: "What are you going to do, Maggie?" '

She looks at me. 'So. I took him to a mental-health wing in a hospital and I left him there. I left him.' Tears run down her cheeks. 'I saw him go downhill. He didn't need a nappy, but they put one on him anyway. It was degrading.' Then he was put in a secure wing in a care home, but he attacked an old woman and they wouldn't let him stay. Then another spell in hospital, then out again into another home, where he stayed for three years. And he always wanted to go home, whatever home was by then, but he couldn't escape. He walked and he walked in the garden, and then one day he fell and he could no longer walk or try to escape or go home to a time when he was safe, a violin tucked under his chin, music flowing through him.

He loved Bach and Beethoven and was obsessed with Beethoven's Opus 131: by the end the score was a 'shattered copy' that he fingered every day. He loved Mendelssohn's violin concerto, and still played it – tried to play it – when he was in the home. Their shared dream had been to convert the old chapel they'd bought into a small concert hall – and now Maggie has done that in his memory, selling his precious violin to raise the money. She sits in the lovely home they once lived in together; in the garden are old gravestones that she tends, though the names of the dead are worn away or mossed over. She remembers her husband and is full of sadness: the man who tried to go home.

William Utermohlen went into the Princess Louise nursing home in 2004. He had stopped painting or drawing. He was incontinent. Although in his self-portraits he looks like a small man, he was over six foot. He kept falling and Pat couldn't pick him up. She could no longer cope. 'I felt dreadful when I let him go. Dreadful and cruel,' she says, not letting herself off the hook. In the photographs of him at the home he stands among the jostle of other residents but the sense of his loneliness is palpable. He is tall, taller than anyone else in the room, and stooped. He never smiles. He looks shockingly sad, existentially alone.

After years of violence and disorder Jan Bell is contented in the home where she now lives. There is order, calm, a sense of being on solid ground at last.

And for Jenni Dutton, 'The care home wasn't a difficult decision at all.' Her mother was becoming increasingly disoriented, and it was time. 'There was lots of music there, reggae – Mum loved reggae – and Ella Fitzgerald, *not* Vera Lynn and the war, which is what they often play. I would walk in and they would all be dancing. I became part of the unit. I looked after people; we'd chat. It was such *fun*. They taught me how to deal with what was happening. You have to go in positively. I had no family with me and I was quite free. I'd go in at all sorts of times; sometimes at eight or nine at night. Everyone who worked there was lovely – simply amazing! It was a home and I was a member of the family.' She looks at me shrewdly. 'I'm not a perfect person, you know. I was getting a great deal out of it.'

This sense of reciprocity is woven through Jenni Dutton's story of caring for her mother. We are often told we have to enter the world of people with dementia, and that is useful advice – but we should also remember that they have something to teach us. Even when the dementia is advanced, there can be reciprocity. These people have lived longer than most and they have the best stories, the most knowledge. Their memory might be failing but their human value remains intact. There is absolutely nothing dutiful or martyred about Jenni Dutton's account of her mother's final years. She talks about them with joy, and with the sense of having received a gift as well as given one. They collaborated together on the 'Darnings', her mother sitting very still while her daughter picked out her image with thread or telling her if she'd got something wrong. And during her mother's years at the home this involvement continued. Even when she was lying in bed, five stone, frail as a bird in winter, Jenni Dutton would sit beside her mother, seeing how the light fell on her face, holding her hand, sometimes taking pictures. She shows me one of these photographs, her mother's head on the pillow, her eyes closed; she could be dead. It's so mercilessly tender and intimate that I almost have to look away, which she notices: 'I did have to stop and ask myself it this was right.' I look at the 'Darnings' hung on the walls around us; the repeated face ageing and unravelling until it is the face of a ghost. 'But old people often look sad, you know,' says Jenni Dutton, reading my thoughts. 'Their muscles relax and sag. We project things on to them.'

She was in it until the end with her mother: daughter, carer, collaborator, recorder of a life that was gently fading. 'I knew from the outset I must have nothing to regret – I guess there's a self-consciousness about that.' That home was home for her mother for a while, or she made it so.

The desire to go home lies very deep in us: it's our place of self-belonging. Odysseus is striving to return to where his wife, Penelope, waits and sews and unpicks the threads, and where his ancient dog will lift its head and recognize him, although to everyone else he is a stranger. Leopold Bloom in James Joyce's retelling of the myth is attempting to go home, wandering through the labyrinths and perils of Dublin. Dorothy in *The Wizard of Oz* travels through witchy lands, along yellow roads, in order to get back to Kansas, at last learning that 'there's no place like home, there's no place like home'. T. S. Eliot's *Four Quartets* weaves itself around this urgent need to be centred in a time, a place and a self: 'We shall not cease from exploration / And the end of all our exploring / Will be to arrive where we started / And know the place for the first time.'

When people in homes try to go home it must be because they no longer feel at home in their lives. In their lostness, they suffer a 'searing' homesickness for the site of 'psychic security'. This sense of absence causes feelings of 'abandonment and dread', like an infant registering the loss of the maternal presence. Apparently, when men feel homesick, it is most often for where they were born and for the comfort of the woman who bore them (all those soldiers who die calling out for their mother). But women who are mothers themselves yearn for that time when their own children were born.

My father loved home. Although his most vivid memories in his dementia years were of being carefree and unattached, in unfamiliar places (evacuated during the war, being in Finland as a young man, national service in Egypt, the heady days of university), he was a homebody. My mother is an adventurer and explorer at heart, often restless, but my father loved returning to his place of safety. Above all, he loved his garden: planting, weeding, pruning, making bonfires, identifying insects and wildflowers, watching small brown birds in the undergrowth, getting his hands dirty. If we ever rented a holiday house, he would make a compost heap there. In many of my childhood memories he is a toiling figure seen through the window, sinking a spade into the soil or gazing intently at something I can't see. His garden was the centre of his home.

In his dementia years, the familiarity of home was increasingly important: everything in its right place, everything known, the shape of the day a comforting repetition, the clock on the wall showing the time, the flowers and plants outside marking the seasons. A few years before my father died, my parents moved from the house they had lived in for three decades in order to be in the middle of a town, where they could walk to the shops and the doctor's. The move itself was a ferocious upheaval – weeks and months of going through possessions that had accumulated over a lifetime. Like many people of their generation, they were thrifty and neither did they throw anything away. My father had about eighty or ninety ties, many faded and fraying. My mother had kept the inner soles of discarded shoes (I remember learning at her funeral that one of my aunts had kept dozens of looped hems that she had cut off from trousers that were too long for her short frame), and Tupperwares that no longer had tops. There were boxes of glasses in the cellar, rolls of moth-eaten carpet in the attic, battered biscuit tins that brought memories of oat cookies and ginger cake flooding back, piles of letters and papers and twenty-year-old bills and plant catalogues from years ago. Chipped china, plates they had bought on their honeymoon in France, tapestry comb cases we had stitched in school when we were little, photos of people whose names they could no longer remember. We found a card my father wrote to my mother: 'To Pat, a short word meaning home.'

In the attic, my sister discovered a canister in which was a reel of film. She took it to be converted into a DVD, and the following Christmas, when my parents were between homes and living with each of us in turn, the extended family gathered to watch it. None of us had any idea what we would see. After a splutter of light and sound, the jerky lines resolved. There was a black-and-white image of a small English church. There were men in suits and women in calf-length dresses and pork-pie hats standing by its porched gate. The church door opened and down the path came a couple, he in a morning suit and she in a wedding dress with a foaming train. A radiant pair, so young and so untried. My mother had her hand tucked into my father's arm and they were both smiling. Smiling at each other and smiling at us, who are waiting for them down the ladder of years. They walked towards us out of the past, radiant with hope for the future. We received them in an anguish of love.

My father's dementia was quite advanced before he left home for a few weeks, to have his leg ulcers healed. (If we could turn back time.) He came back a month later, but he never came home. He never came home to himself.

10. The Later Stages

'I'm all these words, all these strangers, this dust of words, with no ground for their settling, no sky for their dispersing . . .'

Looking back, I think I was strangely acquiescent during my father's long drift, or at least a touch unfocused. It happened so gradually, in those barely discernible, incremental changes that sneak up, Grandmother's Footsteps in the mind, and you don't even know that's the game you're playing. And I was busy, had four children myself, was working hard, blah blah; the excuses we make. Only later, backlit by the trauma of his last months, did I see his decline with any clarity. *So that's what was happening; that's where he was going.* I want to ask him what it felt like; I want to hold his hand and tell him we're all here with him and it will be all right (which of course it won't be, it wasn't). Or just sit in the garden together as the sun goes down.

There came a point when my father was no longer living with dementia but dying with it. And it wasn't a blurred line he softly crossed, it was an abrupt and unignorable rupture – like someone who has been very slowly falling through water suddenly plummeting like a stone, nothing to stop him. To cut a short story even shorter: he went into hospital for treatment that was routine but that he badly needed, and for all sorts of complex reasons got stuck there for five weeks. During that time (I'm wincing as I write this) he was very often quite alone.

The hospital had rigorously enforced visiting hours and then an outbreak of norovirus, so that for many days on end visitors were not allowed in at all. (The category of visitor in this case included the family and carers.) The nurses did their job of nursing, in a ward that, though general, was largely made up of people with dementia and where many patients required a level of attention they could not possibly receive from hard-pressed hospital staff. The doctors doctored. My father, who was a very polite man, lay quietly in his bed. He didn't eat, he didn't drink, he didn't walk or talk or smile into the smiling face of someone who loved him. No one held his hand and read him poetry. If someone had asked him how he was, I'm sure he would have genially said: *Very well, thank you* (until the day when he couldn't find the words to answer).

It was February 2014, a time of storms and floods. The river near my parents' house grew monstrous and flooded into roads and fields. There were swans on the cricket pitch. One time, driving back from the hospital, I saw a man standing on the parapet of the main bridge, police all around him, trying to persuade him not to jump, and water rushing past just beneath him. The sky was like a bruise. Everything felt wild.

My father came home at last, skeletal, immobile, inarticulate and helpless. But he never went upstairs again, or walked in his garden, or danced with my mother, or seasoned the gravy, or teased his grandchildren, or lifted a glass of red wine: *your good health.* I'm a middle-class, middle-aged professional woman; a writer and a journalist. I come from a family of doctors (my father, my brother, one daughter, one nephew, a brother-in-law . . .). I'm impatient, reasonably assertive and don't mind challenging rules – Sean would say I like to. For better or for worse, quite often for worse, I tend to charge into situations where I think I see unfairness or when my blood is up. I find it much easier to act impulsively than to wait things out: I don't bite my tongue, I don't count to ten and I don't let sleeping dogs lie. Why was I so blind and so obedient to the rules? I still don't understand.

In December 2014 I launched a campaign, together with my good friend Julia Jones. It was named after my father. John's Campaign has a very simple principle: that the carers of people with dementia should have the same right to accompany them in hospital as parents do with their sick children; that people with dementia have the right to be so accompanied. It seems unimaginable now that, not long ago, parents were not allowed to be with their children; soon it will seem unimaginable that in many hospitals carers are allowed in only during strictly enforced visiting hours.

John's Campaign, born in the UK, is relevant everywhere, because hospital, *everywhere*, is hazardous for people who are old, frail and confused. The healthcare model in most countries is one of heroic intervention: a tumour removed, a heart set beating again, a leg mended . . . Hospitals are closed, medicalized spaces full of experts, machines, rules. But today, with an ageing population who often have multiple medical conditions and who may get stuck in hospital for months, this model is insufficient. A patient is also a person, valuable and precious and precarious; an infection may be cured and a life wrecked. We are embodied minds in a world charged with intricate connections, webs of belonging and recognition.

Human beings are social beings – and we require social interaction, not just for contentment but for actual function and for survival. Put a person in solitary confinement for a few weeks and they will start displaying signs of mental disturbance. In an article for the *New Yorker*, Atul Gawande asks if the solitary confinement that tens of thousands of prison inmates endure in the US amounts to a form of torture. He cites the work of Harry Harlow, a psychology professor at the University of Wisconsin, who studied the baby rhesus monkey. His most influential, controversial study was on the effect of these monkeys being separated from their mother but, in a later study, he examined the effect of total isolation.

> The researchers found that the test monkeys, upon being released into a group of ordinary monkeys, 'usually go into a state of emotional shock, characterized by . . . autistic self-clutching and rocking'. Harlow noted, 'One of six monkeys isolated for three months refused to eat after release and died five days later.' After several weeks in the company of other monkeys, most of them adjusted – but not those who had been isolated for longer periods. 'Twelve months of isolation almost obliterated the animals socially,' Harlow wrote. They became permanently withdrawn, and they lived as outcasts – regularly set upon, as if inviting abuse.

These are monkeys, of course, not people, and they are babies, not adults. But Gawande believes that what is happening inside American supermax facilities amounts to a similar kind of experiment on adult humans, and we know enough by now to recognize this kind of social deprivation as a cruel, and cruelly effective, kind of torture: it sends many people out of their minds.

There is confirmation of this experiment inside British prisons, where a combination of harsh sentencing policies and an ageing population mean that they have become the largest provider of residential care for frail, elderly people. Because of multiple factors, including lifestyle, availability of drugs and prolonged social isolation, prisoners age much more quickly than other people – they are about fifteen years ahead of the rest of the population, old at sixty-five. Cognitive impairment comes earlier and largely goes undiagnosed and uncared for. Dementia flourishes, unchecked.

In many hospitals, places of healing and rescue, there is an inevitable social isolation that is dangerous for a person whose grip upon the world is already fragile. Put someone with dementia in hospital for a few weeks, wake them at six in the morning with food they don't like, call them by a name they don't recognize (or 'dear' or 'love' or 'we') or don't speak to them much at all, rattle past them with trolleys, push pills into their mouth, rush them in a wheelchair down an endless windowless corridor, wrap tourniquets round their arms, put needles into their skin, stand at the bottom of their bed with several other strangers in white coats or green scrubs and stare at them and write things down with a frown, take away everything that is familiar to them, pull the props of routine from under them, put them in a nappy just in case, deprive them of the people who care for them and understand their needs and speak their language – and they will suffer. Suffer and deteriorate and fall away from their old self and very often never recover. In the UK, one in three people with dementia who go into hospital from home never return home.

In the few weeks after we launched John's Campaign we received hundreds and thousands of messages from carers saying: This happened to us too, to my father, mother, husband, wife, partner, friend. The stories that people have shared from all over the world, and the community of suffering and of goodness they reveal, ring multiple variations on the same theme: their spouses, their parents, were broken, often beyond repair, by their stay in hospital. The eighty-four-year-old wife who had to travel by taxi to visit her husband for the two-hour slot and who wasn't allowed to stay for Christmas dinner; the son battling to keep his frail mother out of hospital after his demented father died there; the patient who lost 30 kilos in six weeks; the daughter whose father was in hospital for fourteen weeks ('four bare walls and a sink'), where 'the plug was pulled' on his life. This life was wrecked; this heartbreak was played out in the very place that was meant to rescue them. The nurses and doctors and hospital staff are almost always diligent, clever and kind – and working for their patients beyond what duty requires. But they cannot possibly give the patient with dementia what they need, which is that intimate connection to the outside world. Stories poured in, full of anger, guilt, powerlessness and loss, countered by ones of encouragement, optimism and advice, and they are still coming.

At the Tavistock Centre, Claire Kent talked of the existential loneliness people can feel while in hospital: 'It's like being by yourself in the dark,' she said. 'It must feel a bit like dying, something you have to do alone.' All the things that keep a person tethered to the life they love may fray and break.

We started the campaign in a kitchen, two middle-aged women saying: *It shouldn't have to be like this*. My father was a few weeks dead and we had only just had his funeral. Julia's mother, June, is in her nineties, with dementia, often chaotic, angry and scared; Julia has always been determined that, should her mother go into hospital, she would accompany her. I find it hard to remember the first months of the campaign with any clarity. I was in a state of distress and also a bit dazed. (I have a vague memory of going on *Woman's Hour* at the time to talk about the novel I'd written, *The Twilight Hour*, which is about a very old woman who is looking back at her life as she moves towards death. I have a recollection of speaking very fast in a strained, emotional voice; everything meant too much; everything was charged with significance.)

I said to someone (actually, I probably said to lots and lots of people, collaring them like a harrowed Ancient Mariner) shortly after my father died that now we could recover him: remember him as he was before the illness took hold of him. But with the campaign I see that I was *literally* trying to recover him. By changing the culture of hospitals, so that the confused and frail didn't go there without their familiars, then I could help him. I was trying to be a saviour; I was trying to atone. I was insomniac, not eating much, fizzing with energy, a bit obsessive. I was insensitive to the feelings of my adored siblings. I wrote an impassioned piece in the *Observer* (the paper where I had worked for many years and which became the hub for the campaign, and without which we could have done nothing). I went on the *Andrew Marr Show* and leaned towards him and waved my hands in the air, while David Cameron, still Prime Minister then, looked on. I went on radio programmes, where it would take a single introductory question to set me off on my emotional tirade. I talked and I wrote about the hidden tragedies that were unfolding in hospital wards up and down the country. We visited the Alzheimer's Society, where I spoke of our campaign as a small, unencumbered rocket. I felt like a rocket, whooshing about on a backthrust of loss and hope. I cycled everywhere, helmet-less, soaked by the rain, masochistic, self-punitive. We went to the House of Commons to talk to ministers. We sat in lots of offices, and kind men and women listened and some of them helped. Looking back at the pieces I wrote over the first few months of the campaign, I see they are full of words like 'kindness', 'compassion', 'moral decency', 'loss', 'tragedy', 'hope'.

Luckily for sore, wonky me, there was Julia, pragmatic and

steadfast. And luckily for us, there were the carers, the nurses, the doctors, the organizers, the people who worked for charities, the managers, the doers and the thinkers who showed us the way to go, introduced us to the right people, advised us, encouraged us, joined us. 'Be kind, for everyone you meet is fighting a hard battle.' Over that year, I became freshly aware both of this great battle we fight and of the kindness of people that runs like an underground river beneath the noise and hurtle of public events. And yet change – even change from which everyone benefits – is hard and slow. I had an image in my mind of a door: pulled open from the inside by the professionals; pushed at from the outside by the carers. Take those doors off their hinges. Let us in. 'Us' is the crucial word, and 'we'. Too many people battle and suffer alone.

In the first year of the campaign we learned what we should have known anyway: there is no magic key. We expected resistance from hospitals and experts and were ready to counter them. Costs: there aren't any, unless hospitals choose, for instance, to put a reclining chair by the bed or subsidize parking, while the benefits are vast. Health and safety: they do it in children's wards and in other countries. The carers' need for respite: this is a right, not a duty; carers may be in great need of respite themselves and should not be made to feel a moral obligation to stay with the patient. The plight of patients without carers: the nurses will be able to give them more time. But in fact, we have met only help and encouragement. We have found there are many tireless groups and individuals who have similar aims to us. Indomitable, humane senior nurses have backed us and shown us examples of enlightened practice, where old, frightened people are treated with respect and humanity. But while people are kind, fragmented, rule-bound systems can grind you down and change comes painfully slowly.

At a Carers UK reception, the chief executive gave me a piece of paper on which she had written down this quotation from the anthropologist Margaret Mead: 'Never doubt that a small group of thoughtful, committed citizens can change the world; indeed, it's the only thing that ever has.' At the time of writing, every acute hospital in England has made a commitment to John's Campaign. There are John's Campaign posters on the doors of hundreds of wards saying the carers are welcome. There are passports for carers. John's Campaign is part of the national audit for dementia. We work with Age UK to implement the campaign across the country. We talk at conferences, produce leaflets, sit on committees. We travel to other countries and take part in the international debate about hospital culture and end-of-life care. But this campaign is the thin edge of a wedge – or maybe it's a Trojan horse. We've never been paid, we've never had a staff (though sometimes people call up and ask to speak to my PA) and we've never had any bureaucracy. We're not a company, not an organization; we're a tiny movement that's part of a larger, worldwide movement for change.

The culture is already transforming – and fast. In the old days (not so long ago or so old) dementia was barely recognized. Andrew Balfour tells me that when he started working as a clinical psychologist he was 'appalled' at how people with dementia were treated. 'It was very distressing. It wasn't that people were deliberately nasty or cruel, but dementia was invisible in those days. As a young man I'd never heard of it!' In those hospitals, 'there was a wiping out of meaning, and of the sense that people's communications were meaningful. It felt like a premature foreclosure of meaning that is an enactment of the illness: a social death of meaning.' He remembers some of those hospitals being 'like Bedlam'. Some people had been in hospital for most of their adult lives with mental illnesses, and now they had dementia too and 'they were warehoused'.

He tells me of an incident that was revelatory for him. One of his patients was an old woman who was always standing up and screaming. Everyone on the ward found her 'very irritating, very grating'. 'I said to her, "You seem very angry," and she replied, "I'm frightened, fucked up and far from home."'

Frightened, fucked up and far from home: I think of all the men and women I've seen lying in their hospital beds, crying out, moaning, obviously frightened but without the words to say of what. Wanting, but not able to say what they want, need, hope for, must have. We don't understand their language. Maybe we have to listen harder and learn it better.

Fifteen months after my father died Sean and I were with my mother in the north of France. It was our first evening there; we'd unloaded the car and stocked the fridge, and now we were sitting in a small, dimly lit brasserie. My mother had a plate of garlicky snails in front of her. She was talking about the day and suddenly she stopped talking; a puzzled expression slid across her face. Her mouth twisted and then she fell against me, her head tipped back, her eyes opened and rolled back, and her whole body slumped: a dead weight – and we did think she was dead. She didn't seem to be breathing.

In the ambulance, she briefly came to and I promised I wouldn't leave. When we arrived at the hospital I ran after the paramedics as they sped her towards the emergency room. But the double doors shut against me and I couldn't get in. I hammered on them and shouted in my rusty French. If she was dying, I needed to be with her. I could feel the panic sharp under my ribs. Eventually I was admitted and led to her bed, where she lay, a tiny figure barely disturbing the sheets, with drips and tubes attached to her, eyes closed but breathing in long, shallow gasps. After a few minutes the nurse told me I could come back in the morning; I said I had to stay. A more senior nurse was summoned and told me to leave; I said I wouldn't. A doctor arrived and said that there were rules: I could return later. I said, 'Non.' In spite of the fact that by this time I was running a campaign in the UK about open access to carers, it felt hard to stand my ground, and perhaps it wasn't even necessary. I was fighting the battle I had lost without even a struggle many months ago. But I'd promised. I could feel my emotions rising in me like a great howl. I couldn't leave (because I had).

There was a French shrug, a long frown of disapproval. I could see myself through his eyes, a dishevelled, hyperbolic, out-of-place woman with a chipped tooth and bags under her eyes. I stayed the night, on a stool, falling asleep and lurching awake through the small hours, listening to my mother breathing. Being there.

I have learned many things during the years of running the campaign – acronyms and bureaucratic structures, train timetables to destinations I never would otherwise have visited, how to read audits, nutritional information, statistics about dehydration and hospital falls and lengths of stay.

Above all, I've learned how lonely it is just to be *I*; how uplifting and consoling to be part of a *we*. Alone, I can do little; together, we can do a great deal.

And I've learned what of course I knew but somehow didn't, that I can't turn back the clock and recover my father, bring him home unbroken. But we can rescue others, as we would wish to be rescued in our turn.

11. Hospitals

In hospitals, time is measured in many different ways. There are clocks on the walls of wards; fob watches tucked inside nurses' pockets, the machines at the head of the bed and the sonar pulse of a heartbeat. The myriad of routines measure off the minutes and the hours; a day is divided up in a rigidly complicated timetable. The lights stutter on in the early morning, the trolleys rattle along corridors which seem to stretch for miles; breakfast, bathroom, bloods, drugs, thermometers, therapies, ward rounds, lunch, visiting hours, menus handed out and filled in, discharge forms, coffee (milky), tea (often tepid), toast, monitoring, maybe visiting time again, supper (very early), meds, bathroom, the lights flicker overhead, machines bleep, and even when the rooms are dimmed and people are sleeping or trying to sleep, the ward rounds continue, people's voices, an emergency somewhere, feet clicking on the linoleum through the night which never really comes, which is endless.

Time is everywhere in a hospital, and inescapable, a bureaucracy in which the patients have little or no control. But it also becomes something unreal and mechanical. It's never dark and never still and never silent. The circadian rhythms of sleep are banished. Morning seeps into afternoon into evening into night. It's a bit like being in transit in an airport terminal, life put on hold, and you could be anywhere, any time, anyone. A body in a bed. An object being processed. Waiting in the small hours, waiting in the dead time, always waiting.

Time can be a tyrant; timelessness a torment. People with

dementia often stay in hospital for many weeks, or even months. My father was there for five weeks, lying in his bed, white hair on his pillow, hyper slow-motion wreckage, smiling genially at the nurses. The calendar in his head quite gone, days gone and seasons gone, at last adrift on the formless sea of time. Tick tock. Time running out. Clangs the bell.

There are large clocks in the flagship ward run by Rowan Harwood, professor of geriatric medicine at Nottingham University Hospital, whose work on providing dignified and compassionate care to his patients with dementia has been something of an inspiration to me. They show the time, the date. I wish my father had come here. It's bright, spotlessly clean, freshly painted, spacious. Each eight-bed area is painted a different colour. There are photos beside every bed. Everything is clearly signed. There are activity areas, social eating, therapeutic interventions. Carers are welcomed and treated as part of the team of support. In this calm, bright space, distress, apathy and even violence are seen as efforts to communicate.

At Sussex University medical and nursing students are paired with a person with dementia and their family so that they can gain insight into what it is to be old and become interested in a humane way in an illness that they will almost certainly encounter in their career. The patients become their mentors. 'Our job,' says Sube Banerjee, 'is to create the next generation who are a bit less rubbish than we are.'

Hospital after hospital, up and down the country: I wish I could name them all and the people who work there, my roll call of gratitude. There are art classes, music sessions, volunteers who come to do patients' hair for them, paint their toenails, give them hand massages, thumb through photo albums, hand out tea. There are 'This is Me' booklets at the end of beds, so that while the patient might be unable to articulate their own likes and dislikes, they are written down clearly (what name they want to be called by, who their family members are, what food they love or hate, what their interests are, what their job once was, where they lived as a child, what makes them them). There are charities that bring in dogs and other animals. That make twiddlemuffs – knitted comforters that people with dementia often find it reassuring to hold and fiddle with. Rooms for carers who want to stay the night. Rooms for the dying. (Most people don't want to die in hospital and most people do.)

In one hospital, a nurse tells me about the man with dementia who doesn't have any visitors and who has just spent his eightieth birthday there. No one visits him. The nurses asked him what he most wanted and he told them that when he was a boy his favourite treat was the treacle tart his mother used to make. They bought him one from a shop down the road, put candles on it, and nurses, carers and other patients gathered round to sing 'Happy Birthday' to him. He wept; everyone else wept; I nearly wept when I heard the story. Small acts of intimate, daily kindness that revive the sense of collective humanity and of the enduring self.

I spend the day with Jo, the dementia lead at a large hospital trust, and her colleagues Lucy and Aishlene. Jo was one of the first people to contact us about John's Campaign, and calmly, quietly, resolutely, she has put the principle of welcome for carers into practice across every ward in all the hospitals in the trust. Self-deprecating and humorous, she is an invincible champion for people who live with dementia. In the hours that I am with them, in their office, on their rounds, I learn something of what their job entails. It is both simple and painfully, complicatedly hard.

Rowan Harwood – the Nottingham professor – once genially rebuked me, saying, 'There's more to it than just being
kind, you know,' yet in a sense, what I witnessed all through
that optimistic day was precisely kindness. But kindness isn't
easy; it's never *just* kindness. It involves a scrupulous vigilance
to individual needs; a nimble, improvisatory imagination; a
common-sense and patient determination to find the unique
and precious person who may be obscured by their dementia.
The team's job is one of hope (which is also how Sube Banerjee
describes his). They believe that their patients are legible
beings and, however confused and chaotic, however violent or
passive or apparently incoherent, they possess a meaning and
a self. Jo and her team always have faith that they can crack
a person's code and find their way through the apparently
impassable muddle and distress to reach them. A large part of
their job is to understand each patient as an individual, with
a long history, a set of relationships, unique needs and desires.
Jo calls herself, Aishlene and Lucy 'investigators': they find
out the person's work, family, interests, likes, favourite foods,
any of the triggers that might bring them back. This bringing-
back can seem miraculous – like someone returning from the
underworld.

'We are on the side of the patient,' Jo says. 'You have to learn
to understand what they are telling you. Nobody can say
our patients don't communicate. Oh, they communicate! They
might not be able to use words, but they can throw things,
spray water over the nurses, shout. They don't lose their self,
just their ability to communicate. They still have feelings,
they still have stories. They are still there. They partly can't
communicate that, and they partly can't conceal it.' This sense
of being both hidden and exposed makes them very complex
as patients, and the task of Jo and her team is intricate and

subtle. 'And *fun*,' adds Jo. 'They're more interesting than most patients and you have to be able to have fun; you have to love difference.'

I go round the wards with Aishlene. We talk to patients, take their hands, look at their photos, meet their relatives. Aishlene gives them pictures she has printed out. A cricket team. Flowers. A familiar face. One of them loves reggae, and she puts on music; he half dances in his chair, shuffling his feet on the floor.

Then we sit high up in the labyrinthine hospital, in the small room that is the headquarters of their investigations. Several desks and computers have been inserted into the small space. The shelves are crammed with squeezy pigs, squashy balls, aroma stones, soft toys and twiddlemuffs. The kettle boils. The phone rings constantly – relatives who want advice and reassurance. They tell me stories about their patients and I'm struck by how they *like* them, taking enormous pleasure in their eccentricities and difficult behaviour. Even their rudeness and violence are seen as symptoms that they can, with ingenuity and imagination, resolve.

The stories they tell are ones of salvage: a man who was continually agitated is now calm because they can show him picture books that will take him back to his past. The couple who cared for each other devotedly and who were admitted to hospital together when the husband was in his last days so they need not be separated. Another couple who died within a day of each other, the husband lying beside his wife as she breathed her last, and then it was his turn. The severely depressed patient who felt he was in prison there and so they wrapped him up, put him in a wheelchair and took him into the streets. ('You should have seen his face: he was in awe of the air!')

The woman who was always crying out and distressed. Her

family said that it was normal: she was always like that. 'It's not normal to be always agitated. She was telling us something. Eventually we discovered that the woman had arthritis and it was uncontrolled pain that was making her so upset. We have given her pain patches and now she's out in the corridor, playing bowls.'

Or the man with seventeen adored grandchildren who found great solace in the baby dolls that Jo and her team gave to him to look after.

The woman with red glasses, one lens missing, cursing like a trooper and no way that anyone is going to tell her what to do, using her soft-toy dog like a whip.

The woman who had never been seen naked, even by her own husband, with whom she'd had three children: 'She was refusing to have a shower and no wonder. At the very least, she shouldn't have a male nurse.'

The man who loved numbers and was very agitated: 'We gave him sums, which we had deliberately got wrong, to mark.' The woman – stick-thin and floridly psychotic – who thought Tony Blair was trying to kill her. She would spend her time crouched under the nursing station, taking cover. 'She was very religious so we took her to the chapel where she had a rapturous evangelical moment, crying out: "Praise be to God, and where am I?" '

People with dementia, they tell me, never do what you expect. 'You have to go in at a deeper level. You have to think outside the box. And then, just to see the difference – any difference. To see someone smiling when you've been told they never smile. Just to get some of what is left inside.'

So there they go, walking down the corridor with a photo album, a bottle of wine, a zoo of soft animals and twiddle-muffs, with hope and determination. The investigators.

'Dementia is *hideous* if it's managed badly,' says Jo. 'But it needn't be hideous.'

I left the hospital feeling moved but also strangely exhausted, like there was a thick sludge under the brightness. Optimism in the face of so much distress and disorder is a tiring business, a question of will and endurance: never to give up.

There is still a self, Jo says. They are still here.

It is possible for a hospital to be a place of safety and kindness for a person who is frail and confused and full of fear, where a patient is also protected as a person, cherished as a human, and where their sense of self is rediscovered and salvaged. But – to state the bleeding obvious – it is often not like this. It can be a place where a precarious sense of self is finally extinguished and the social being is obliterated.

No matter how resourceful and kind the nurses are, how good and clear-sighted the doctors, the needs of an individual can be easily lost in the vast, intricate mechanics of healthcare. Rules that grow up for good reasons become muscle-bound and intractable; effective management can harden into sclerotic bureaucracy. Staff are pinned to their work stations by computers and forms and boxes to tick. There are drugs and operations and meals and regimes and machines beside each bed; there are crises that trigger swift medical responses – and all the while, the slow-motion crisis of a mind in the process of being picked apart goes on silently, invisibly, in hundreds and thousands of bays: men and women living become men and women dying. Going and going and gone.

To have dementia 'is physiological, it's psychological, it's social,' says Sube Banerjee. 'It doesn't fit into the structures we've created. We've got to think complex. We've got to change the culture. We've got to know what good looks like; it's *our* business, everyone's. And the perfect time is always now.'

Hospitals have traditionally been places of cure. Sometimes people can't be cured. They can be cared for, recognized, seen not just as bodies but as embodied minds. In every country, it is increasingly understood by healthcare staff that hospitals are hazardous places to be for people with dementia. Huge efforts are being made to reduce the risk they pose (which is where John's Campaign comes in). But the wheels of change turn slowly and, in the meantime, intimate tragedies unfold.

12. *At the End*

'We possess art lest we perish of the truth.'

I used to see an old man in shabby clothes standing at the busy junction near our house in north London. He held in his hand a piece of cutlery (usually a fork, I think), which he waved high in the air as the cars and buses roared by, sometimes with enormous energy and sometimes quite calmly.

He didn't seem unhappy, but he was certainly a solitary figure, unaware of the people who passed him by. He was in his own world. I assumed – rightly – that he had dementia. Then he disappeared. The obituaries that followed revealed that he had been a psychoanalyst and brilliant musicologist whose research had added significantly to our knowledge of how Beethoven and Mozart composed their music. Only then did it occur to me that perhaps with his fork, his spoon, he had been conducting the traffic to the music in his head. This image has always haunted me because of the great disconnect between what we all saw – a demented old man weaving around on the pavement – and what he was experiencing, which I like to imagine was both the music of the composers he had so loved and also a sense of centrality and of control over his world.

No one comes back from the land of advanced dementia to tell us what it is like there. Like the pulsing light on a sonar screen, they dim until they can no longer be traced, and we can't imagine what they are experiencing, there in the cold, deep darkness. The old woman lying in bed next to my daughter, who shouted the same terrified words over and over again: was she vividly experiencing a past trauma or had her mind simply snagged on a stump of memory and stuck there? The woman who stumbled towards me at the care home, repeating: 'Hymns of comfort, hymns of comfort' – was she distressed, or were the words separated from any meaning? When my father joined in with 'I must go down to the seas again', I have no idea if he was seeing in his mind the spume flung off waves, the sea mist and the white sails shaking, or if these words were traces, just the last random sparks thrown out by a dying mind.

To think about the final stages of dementia is to think about what it is to be human, and it is to acknowledge the essential loneliness and separation of the individual mind. We spend our lives forging relationships with others, trying to imagine ourselves into their lives, trying to communicate our own feelings – throwing frail bridges across the great divide of self from self. To fall in love is to believe that we can be known, *truly* known, by someone else, and that we can in turn know them, feel with them, and through overwhelming attachment and desire merge: two stories streaming into one. (To fall out of love is to withdraw into the defended self again, to pull up the bridge.) We may reach out, strain towards each other, tell our stories and spill our guts, give secrets as gifts, but we can never enter into the mind of another or know what the world looks like through their eyes, what their particular pain feels like, on the skin or in the heart. In the end, we're mysterious to each other.

Towards the end of my time with Jo and her team of dementia nurses, Jo asked me if I'd seen Gladys. I didn't know what she meant or who Gladys was. She sat down at her computer and searched for the site, then pressed play. The four of us watched the short film that Jo thinks every nurse – and every *person* – should watch. In it, Naomi Feil, founder of Validation Therapy, which began in the US but is now practised all over the world, is shown with Gladys Wilson, a woman with severely advanced dementia who is now unable to speak. Validation Therapy is about communication through empathy, about entering the world of the other. 'Their desperate need for connection is all inside now,' says Naomi Feil. 'If the person is all alone, even if they're very, very deteriorated, there is a longing for this kind of closeness.'

We see Gladys Wilson sitting in a tall-backed chair, fidgeting her fingers on the armrests. There is a crocheted blanket over her lap. Her head is back, her mouth half open to show her two remaining teeth, one eye is shut and it is impossible to tell if she is seeing anything. Naomi Feil approaches her, crouches beside her, calls her by her proper name – Mrs Wilson – and takes her restless hand. Gladys Wilson holds on to Naomi Feil's hand, pulls and shakes at it, rocks back and forth. There is a single tear on the old woman's face and Naomi Feil wipes it away very gently, then strokes Gladys Wilson's face with her fingertips – 'where the mother usually touches an infant' so that 'every cell remembers that touch'. She is 'no longer alone'. Gladys Wilson's eyes are fully open now, and she is staring with a kind of desperate intensity into the face of the woman who is asking her to 'let me in a little bit'. One hand bangs repeatedly on the armrest and her face works. Then Naomi Feil begins to sing to her, 'Jesus, love me' – because she knows that Gladys Wilson has always been very religious. She is still stroking the old woman's face. The banging hand gradually falls into rhythm. When Gladys Wilson moves, so does Naomi Feil, mirroring her; when the banging gets faster, so does the singing, and when it slows so does the song. And then Gladys Wilson pulls the therapist to her so their faces are pressed together, like mother to child. Now, when Naomi Feil sings, Gladys Wilson joins in. 'He's got the whole world in his hands.'

I watch this poignant little film with Jo and her team, and I watch it again when I return home and I watch it once more before writing this. It's beautiful: it recognizes the person trapped inside the failing body and mind and is an act of profound humanity. It's like a trickle of clear water on parched land. It's also terrifying: I can scarcely bear it. What is Gladys Wilson feeling as she clutches at the therapist's hands, leans forward, tears on her cheeks. Joy? Relief? Peace? Utter despair? For a brief moment the old woman is touched, embraced, stroked, crooned to, loved like a tiny child is loved. Then she is let go. She sinks back again in her chair. Her eyes close again and her fingers scrabble at the armrest. I am left with a sense of squeamish disquiet. Was it purely good to briefly rescue her from her existential loneliness, or is it also a kind of torment?

This extraordinary act of recognition reaffirms the humanity not only of the old woman but of the therapist who joins her. We start by seeing Gladys Wilson from a distance, a wrecked, twitching figure in a chair, and we end by looking into her eyes, watching her cry, seeing her as a subject, not an object; a person, not a thing. Naomi Feil treats her with respect (she calls her Mrs Wilson, asks for permission before she comes close and embraces her). Respect means to *look again*. So we look again at Gladys Wilson, and we look again at all the people that we usually look away from: don't see, don't recognize. That man shouting in the street, that woman helpless in the bed, the person slumped in a chair, wearing a nappy, whose head is tipped forward, all those old, frightened, contorted faces that have such power to horrify us. We sometimes talk of people with very advanced dementia as animals or vegetables, precisely because it is much easier than acknowledging that they are one of us. It is painful to accept that we too might become like that, and even if we don't, even if we happen to be one of the lucky ones through no virtue of our own, these old and confused people show us what it is to be mortal, bodily and at the mercy of strangers.

The mystery of what goes on inside the mind of another person becomes terrifyingly impenetrable in the final stages of dementia; twilight to pitch dark at the vanishing line between life and death. Scientists can scan brains and measure damage but they can't show us what it is actually like to be in a world where time has ceased to have any meaning, where the past does not connect to the present and where the present does not lead to an anticipated future. History is lost and expectation has gone and now is all that remains; now and now and now.

Nor can they show us what it is like to have no language left – or the barest scrap, a remembered word or phrase still lodged somewhere in the shattered memory, like a survivor of the wreckage.

(One of my father's carers, in his last months, was French. She said to him one day: *Ça va, John?* And he smiled at her and said, *Ça va très bien, merci* – he must have chanted the phrase when he was a schoolboy sitting at his wooden desk, wearing the words into a groove of memory, and now it came back to him, miraculously finding its way through the self's shattered landscape. Is this memory, or memory's trace?)

Carol Gilligan writes: 'To have a voice is to be human. To have something to say is to be a person. But speaking depends on listening and being heard; it is an intensely relational act.' Gilligan defines voice as 'something like what people mean when they speak of the core of the self', so that 'speaking and listening are forms of psychic breathing'. Home is where they speak your language; loss of language is an exile and a home-sick separation from the self. Words are not like a skin over meaning but like a bucket dipped into a deep well. To speak ourselves is to make a narrative, and this narrative self is what gives us our coherence. We lose words, we lose the plot. Words fail us. At first they drop away individually, like pebbles off the mountain slope. More and more, until the sinister trickle turns into an avalanche of loss, meanings plunging away, a great roar of silence. At what point do we lose ourselves?

There's a crucial distinction between losing the sense of self and losing the self. One of the reasons the philosopher Ronald Dworkin supports those who chose death should they have advanced dementia is that at this point 'they are ignorant of self . . . Because they have no sense of a whole life, a past joined to a future . . .' The value of their life is diminished or even destroyed, because 'value cannot be poured into life from the outside, it must be generated by the person whose life it is, and this is no longer possible'.

Dworkin makes a clear distinction between the inner self and the outer world; he believes that meaning is generated from within. Individuals are their own meaning-generating world. But a person, as Bishop Desmond Tutu has it, depends on other people to be a person. And the philosopher Martin Buber, best known for his philosophy of dialogue, coined the term widely used by ethicists: 'I–Thou'. 'Speech does not reside in man,' he writes, 'but man takes his stand in speech . . . Spirit is not in the *I* but between *I* and *Thou*. It is not like the blood that circulates within you but the air in which you breathe.' So we live in a 'shared space of meaning': language, which puts everything 'out in the open', creates a public space. The mind is not only inner; the boundaries between the inner and outer are porous. 'It is messy and fascinating to be minded people in the world.'

It is this 'I–Thou' that Naomi Feil was entering, or trying to enter, with Gladys Wilson; the air they briefly breathed together. Although the person with advanced dementia cannot form the most basic narratives of daily life and all coherence of the self has gone, although words no longer make sentences, syntax is gone, words for objects lost and one thing no longer follows from another but falls apart in fragments which, like Humpty Dumpty, we cannot put together again, they still precariously exist in this 'I–Thou', in this dream of a common language.

In the 'ruins of grammar', in the 'forever in my mouth/and forgetting', in the 'dirty taste of gone', tiny bubbles of memory and memory traces come winking to the surface. Pronouns are often the last to go. 'You', 'me' and 'I' – that small, vital centre in Tommy Dunne's concentric rings that he pulls up to show me. 'I am.' Until the very last stages there is still an *I* in dementia. The eighteenth-century satirical writer Jonathan Swift anticipated his own psychological deterioration, now widely thought to be dementia, long before it happened ('See how the Dean begins to break . . . That old vertigo that's in his head/ Will never leave him till he's dead . . .'). For him life was a 'dark and desolate farce' and the bulk of his inheritance went to founding an institution for 'as many lunatics and idiots as possible'. The slow loss of his faculties made his final years painful ones; his mind failed, his sight failed, his speech failed until he was barely able to utter a word, and yet in the year before his death, he could say: 'I am what I am, I am what I am,' and the last words he uttered were, apparently, 'I am a fool.'

Gladys Wilson can no longer say, 'I am'; the few words she utters in the film are memory traces: a line of the song she must have sung over and over again.

Jenni Dutton's mother, a tiny figure lying in her bed, probably could not say, 'I am.'

Nor could Rebecca Myer's mother in her final days in the home. She could no longer recognize her husband or her children; she was struggling to swallow. Because Rebecca's father could not bear to take the decision to let her die, they inserted a PEG tube to feed her and keep her going: she wasn't really living, though; she was dying, very slowly dying.

William Utermohlen was also, in those last years in a care home, beyond language – which for him had been the language of art. When he tried to write his own name, the words broke up, the letters toppled into each other. Syllable by syllable, William Utermohlen is disappearing. The laceratingly moving self-portraits are done with now. Over several heroic years he had confronted his own deterioration and portrayed himself as broken, mutilated, his world violently and dizzyingly slipping away from him. In making these works, he was attempting to 'fix an image of the self' and 'calling forth his double', like seeing himself in the mirrors that he became so scared of his wife hung drapes over them. This double is a ghost, or a shadow, or a man so existentially lost that we can hardly bear to meet his gaze. He sees himself with a saw in a premonition of the autopsy that will disclose his wounded brain; through bars; in disintegrating space, with one huge ear, his face dotted over, his nose like a beak, a vanishing object, the lines getting fainter, the world emptying around him and everything that anchored him gone. He erases himself. He is still there, faint lines that fade to white.

He is nearly gone, a scribbled death head with eyes that remain his own, staring out at us from the terrible demolition of the self.

Once people with dementia can no longer speak or communicate, reaching out to us from their darkness, how can we imagine their state or try to alleviate their suffering?

Illness has always been a subject for art and, over the last few years, as the population ages and the number of those who have the illness dramatically increases, dementia has entered our culture and our consciousness so quickly it is hard to keep up. From being hidden and largely invisible, it is at last talked and written about, and the uniquely cruel, distressing and destabilizing nature of its tragedy acknowledged. John Bayley wrote an elegy about Iris Murdoch's loss of memory; Sally Magnusson wrote her groundbreaking book about her beloved mother's dementia; Timothy West has been moving about the Alzheimer's of his wife, the actor Prunella Scales. Terry Pratchett was heroic in his openness about his own dementia, both funny and sad. The floor of my study is piled with accounts by people living with the illness and memoirs by those who cared for them. Harrowing, funny, poignant, harsh, they crack open the locked room. Light floods in where once there was secrecy, shame and terror.

But most of these accounts – shocking, touching, candid, empathetic – are still, inevitably, external. They are often written by people at the start of their illness or by carers, the intimate observers of the process of self-loss. The final stage of dementia thwarts the attempts to describe its internal experience because it is beyond language. Art, however, can try to enter the silent darkness. I can come up with very few dramatizations of dementia before the last fifty or so years. Sometimes

I have wondered if Haydn's 'Farewell' Symphony – in which one by one the musicians lay down their instruments and leave the stage, music gradually thinning into silence – is an evocation of it. There is, of course, the melancholy Jaques's seven-ages-of-man speech in *As You Like It* (starting with the 'infant, mewling and puking' in its nurse's arms and ending with a 'second childishness' of decrepitude: 'sans teeth, sans eyes, sans taste, sans everything'). Or King Lear, who endures a storm that is both literal and psychological, whose identity crumbles and whose words fall away, and who dies. Friends have pointed to the Aged P in Charles Dickens's *Great Expectations*; maybe Mr Wodehouse in Jane Austen's *Emma*; perhaps Don Quixote.

Recently, however, depictions of dementia have become so common in art that they are almost a trope. Films such as the Oscar-winning *Still Alice* have characters with Alzheimer's at their centre, as does the beautiful and heartbreakingly joyful Disney animation *Coco*. But these are all realist texts that remain stable in spite of their subject matter. They can't resist the notion of plot, order, a single coherent self. Dementia might be the subject, but it does not disrupt the narrative, or do away with it. During dementia's end-game, a person goes to a place where we cannot follow them and can barely guess at. The bursts of lucidity that those with catastrophic memory loss can sometimes have are like bright, sharp flashes of lightning over a blasted landscape – or perhaps even that is wishful thinking and they signify nothing at all. We hang on to meaning and insist on it. The child learns to shape sounds into words and make boundaries around things; they tell stories and impose a narrative pattern on to chaos. Only in this way can the flooding world be comprehensible and endurable. But the person with dementia unshapes, undoes, disintegrates, unravels – from the formation of the self and language to its drastic unmaking. Words become mere sound again.

The art that attempts not simply to observe and describe but to *inhabit* that desolate place of self-loss edges us towards that darkness and silence and absence and becomes like an emotional modernism in which there is no central narrator, no coherent story, where things are fractured and the safe ground slides away beneath our feet. Exploring the experience of dementia and the loss of memory can bring about a powerful and vertiginously unsettling way of thinking about time, place and identity, where the notion of a stable reality and a single self breaks apart. It's a de-creation, in which words and meanings are unmade – an apocalypse of the self. Instead of observing the experience of loss from the outside, we who still possess our selves are given the chance to imaginatively enter that world, briefly experiencing its terror and loss.

In 2015 I went to see Florian Zeller's play *The Father* (translated from the French by Christopher Hampton) and was completely winded by the experience. Its central character, who when I saw it was played with gusto and heartbreak by Kenneth Cranham, has Alzheimer's. It starts calmly, with a comfortingly ordinary bourgeois living room: bookshelves, table, armchairs, pictures, an old man talking to his daughter. We realize that he is losing his memory but at first we are simply observing an all-too-familiar family drama. Within minutes we are wrong-footed; the ground gives way. Whose flat are we in – his or hers? Is she his daughter and, if so, who is this other woman who says she too is Anne? Who is the man who says he is Andre's son-in-law, and why are there two of them? Was Andre a dancer or an engineer in his professional life? Why does the dinner of roast chicken keep repeating? Where is his watch? Is time on a nightmarish loop, is it slipping away, or is it more like a cancerous cell dividing and mutating?

We never know the answers because senselessness and terminal confusion are the point ('It doesn't make sense,' says Andre, over and over again). Between short scenes interspersed with increasingly jarred and stuck music the furniture on the stage gradually disappears, just as the furniture of the old man's mind is broken up. In the end there is just a white-sheeted bed in a white-painted room, an old man calling for his mother. Here is the radical slowness of death reaching its end point at last. The audience both inhabits Andre's mind and at the same time tries to decode its erratic signals, for *The Father* – beautifully, heartbreakingly and exhilaratingly – continually reminds us of our need to make a story out of chaos while brutally undercutting it. Like Bernlef's excruciating *Out of Mind*, for example, or like Kazuo Ishiguro's *The Unconsoled*, it evokes the painful struggle with language and the thwarted attempts to communicate that which lies beyond communication, the impossibility of capturing the 'de-wording, de-languaging, de-remembering'.

Language is also memory; dementia brings a double silence. The death of the self is the death of an entire world. Beta-amyloid plaques and tangled brain neurons; lifeless grey patches spreading through glorious colours of the working brain. Words seep away like blood. Hidden people, in that cave where light doesn't reach, and from which no signals return to us. We can only stand at the threshold of the silence, the darkness and the absence.

I think of the people I have known and loved who have spent their last years in the hidden land of dementia from which none return. We come into the world with nothing and gradually we build up the vast, rich palace of the self: language and knowledge and relationships and belongings and experience and memory and love. Above all, memory and love. All these fall away as life returns to that state of nothing. When we cannot even say 'I am.' When we cannot.

Yet still the old man waves his fork into the air. Perhaps he hears music.

13. *Saying Goodbye*

'What is loss? Loss is a sleeping giant.'

My father had retired late, just as his illness was starting to take a grip on him. He didn't have time for the retirement he had planned: working in his garden, wandering in the woods and walkways near their house, tracking butterflies and collecting the seeds of wildflowers, travelling with my mother to Corsica, where they had had many holidays. Instead, he entered a kind of twilight zone, bit by bit slipping away from the life he had planned for; knowing and then mercifully not knowing what he was leaving and what he was losing.

Dementia is a particularly long farewell to the self. With most illnesses, death comes quite swiftly. With dementia, the flicker with which life ends is excruciatingly slowed. People who live with it may have plenty of time to contemplate their own going; their carers have even longer, often many years of imagining and preparing and rehearsing. There's an anticipated, ambiguous grief; a premature mourning of the self, or of the beloved other.

During dementia's last stages, a beloved person may be there and yet absent, a powerful reminder of the self's loss. Dismantled in the drawn-out end-game, yet they remain – like apparitions, haunting us and themselves: the figure in the mirror who they no longer recognize or perhaps recognize as their dead parent, their ghostly other. Of everyone I've talked to, only Patricia Utermohlen said that her husband's real death happened before the actual one, at the point at which he laid down his pencil. This was the vanishing line. Nevertheless, she did not stop visiting him, and nor did his old friend Ronnie Carroll.

Pauline, who describes her mother as 'the living dead', imagines the sadness she will feel when she is finally gone. 'What will I say at her funeral? That she tried to make the best of it. I'm still sad she couldn't do more.'

To mourn someone who is still alive brings a particular, complicated pain. And often it brings guilt: to mourn someone who has not yet died is to consign them to a kind of death.

Disie Johnson gave away her husband's paints. She can't bring herself to give away his beautiful suits, though he will never wear them again.

Rebecca Myers describes the final years of her mother's life as ones of 'mourning'. Her mother died a long fourteen years after her diagnosis. She was struggling to swallow and they put in the PEG tube that kept her alive: 'and once the tube is in that's giving her food, it's very difficult to remove it. It becomes an active decision.'

Shortly after her mother went into the home her father was diagnosed with multiple myeloma, a cancer of the blood. He had to have a marrow transplant and was very sick. At the same time, Rebecca's husband, a GP, was hit by a tipper truck and both of his ankles were crushed. He had multiple surgeries over the following years and lost his practice. There was trouble over the funding of her mother's care, which was judged to be social, not medical. Now they were told they needed to pay £2,000 per month, money they did not have: her father had been spending all his money after his cancer diagnosis (her mother died before their appeal could be heard). They were in a sea of troubles. Rebecca had to return to work. Her mother was at the end-stage; she needed end-of-life care. It was suggested that a DNR should be put in place and nature should take its course – but even now, 'it was a tough decision' and one her father struggled to come to terms with. At last he agreed.

Just before Christmas her father was rushed into hospital with kidney cancer; her mother was rushed into A & E, where she was given antibiotics – 'But why? *Why?* My mother was in hospital; my father was in hospital; my husband was on crutches; and I – well, I was a madwoman.'

Sometimes, we outlive our selves.

Jo and her team of 'investigators' are acutely aware that sometimes people need to be let go. 'If they are at their end,' says Jo, 'we will know from their story.'

She tells me about a Somalian woman who was clearly at the end of her life. She knew it herself: she kept trying to pull out the tubes that were keeping her alive. But her son wasn't ready for her to die. She had been an amazing woman, an amazing mother – and moreover, when she died, he would be the head of the family. 'He needed time,' says Jo. 'So we gave him time.' They kept the tubes in, kept her going, and after a week he returned and said: 'I'm ready.'

'It's really hard to have that conversation. It's really, really hard to say goodbye.'

Research commissioned by the Dying Matters Coalition in the UK in 2018 showed that, of the people interviewed, nearly 70 per cent said they were comfortable with talking about their wishes for end-of-life care with the family, and only 29 per cent had discussed their wishes. And while most people believe it is important to draw up an Advanced Care Plan, only about 10 per cent actually do so.

A survey conducted by the Conversation Project in the US in 2013 demonstrates how this reluctance to talk about dying and death is universal. Nine out of ten Americans believe it's important for them and their loved ones to talk about end-of-life care but only three out of ten have actually had these conversations. The reasons people gave for this were several: they aren't sick yet, the subject makes them uncomfortable, they don't want to upset their family, it's not the right time, they are waiting for someone else to start the conversation . . .

It's difficult to talk about dying, about becoming dead. To mourn is to know what one has lost – but to mourn what one has not yet quite lost is to be in a kind of limbo.

Tommy Dunne says that not a day goes by when he does not grieve for the Tommy Dunne who is no more. 'I've never been scared of dying. If I was told I had three days left to live, I don't think I would be scared. But I'm frightened when I look in the mirror and don't recognize myself. And I miss the Tommy I was.'

Theresa Clarke says that the time will come when she will no longer be in possession of her true self. 'I will do the best I can here for as long as I can. I don't know what it will be like as my memory closes down. But I hope I have enough time to go out on my own terms.' Her eyes are bright, her expression canny. 'I am quite happy to end my life, you know. I have no children. My siblings are all dead or old. I can do it on my own terms. I will see myself out in my own way. I've thought about it – and not in a negative way at all. I'm realistic. I'm not a saint, but I believe I've been a good person. I'm counting on my experience to notice what is changing; I've always had an agile brain. I'll be leaving because I no longer have control in my life or joy in my life. I won't tell anyone. I love life, but I have no fear of dying. Actually' – she put her head on one side in that way she has – 'I am quite looking forward to it. For life is a struggle. I explored. I was nosy. And I want to be aware that I am leaving life. I've seen other people in those last stages – it isn't good. I need to go on my own terms. My mother would say: "That's our Theresa."'

She means it, may likely do it. But it's hard to say goodbye to ourselves.

One of my favourite jokes goes like this: How do you make God laugh? Tell him your plans.

Dementia has become the illness we most fear: and this is a special way of being afraid, not just Philip Larkin's furnace-fear of death but fear of a living death, of a nightmarish incarceration within the decaying body and mind.

I trawl through the advice on how to prevent it. There's a lot of it, some precise and some general, some feasible and some not. Eat raw fruit and vegetables. Exercise. Eat fish. Get a hearing aid. Do crosswords or some such brain-training thing . . .

(There are brain-training sessions you can download: five minutes every day of exercises, starting off simple – as in, here are three words: *hut, hot, spy*; now tell me what's the second letter of the first word, the first letter of the third word, the last letter of the middle word? – and getting more complicated. I quickly get myself in a pickle.)

. . . Learn a new language. Stop smoking. Sleep better. Eat a Mediterranean diet. Take K vitamins. Meditate and be mindful. Think. Run. Communicate. Complete secondary education. Lose weight (if you're overweight). Don't be lonely. Seek help for depression. Sing. Dance. Play an instrument. Walk. Laugh. Connect. Connect. Connect. Only connect.

When I started writing this book I made myself a list of the things that I would do should I discover that I had dementia.

- Put my financial affairs in order and update my will
- Write a living will, stating my precise wishes, including a DNR
- Investigate ways of choosing the time and manner of my death
- Say the diagnosis out loud to everyone I know, taking Tommy and Theresa as my inspirations
- Write a letter to Sean
- Write a letter to each of my four children
- Throw away things I don't want people to find
- Radically tidy my home
- Start giving things away
- Say sorry to a few people who are on my conscience
- Do those things I've always promised myself I would do, one day, when I have time, space, freshness (not one of those bucket lists, but read the great novels that I've missed; revive the disintegrating Italian I used to speak; listen to nightingales sing in the woods near our house)
- Have fun (as the great Dr Seuss says in *The Cat in the Hat*, 'fun is good', but it's strangely easy to forget that)
- Stop hurtling through life in that great race against time we can never win . . .
- Read poetry every day, out loud
- Do more wild swimming
- Dance with abandon

- Avoid self-pity: as Tommy says, Why *not* me?
- Make peace with myself; let go of anger; still my restless heart
- Eat oysters every day

I should probably do most of these things anyway, of course. We shouldn't have to wait for a diagnosis before we attempt to lead a better life. Life is finite from the start – a finite life is a precious one. We will all be mourned in the end.

I think of Theresa Clarke, walking, walking, walking, up and down, and round and round the small room that contains her whole world now. Holding on to herself, waiting for the time when she can no longer . . .

I think of Tommy and the concentric rings that he showed me on his iPad, and of his heroic attempts not to lose the protecting circle that is Joyce, that is love, that is the final circle before he only has the lonely *I*.

Of William Utermohlen making his marks on the canvas: a staring eye, a beak, a white space where once the world burst in.

I think of my father. I think of him smiling at me – 'Hello, Nic' – and am rinsed through with sadness and gladness. When the long trick's over.

To live until we die. If only.

14. Death

'Death twitches. "Live," he says. "I am coming." '

It has become easier to live longer but harder to die well. In previous centuries, death was familiar and not hidden behind institutional walls: before the twentieth century, there would have been scarcely an adult who had not seen their parents, some of their children and their friends die. Moreover, there was faith that it was not the end. People witnessed death, dealt with it, prepared for it, even embraced it; it was public and accepted. Now, although we live with the sense of our own ending, we don't, really. We know we're going to die, but we don't *know*. Our body doesn't know, except in dizzying moments of terror, not until the sentence has been uttered and the gallows are being built under the window.

Even then, death is often held at bay and life prolonged at all costs: the fragile and disintegrating body is plugged into machines, pumped full of oxygen and blood and drugs, its gallant heart restarted and kept going, no matter the pain, no matter the hopelessness of the endeavour, no matter that at a certain point this isn't living, just a slowed-down, drawn-out, painful and undignified dying. Death has become an aggressively medicalized and bureaucratic process placed in the hands of experts; sometimes banal, sometimes farcical, sometimes painful or undignified. Modern, sanitized death becomes a dirty little secret, almost embarrassing: our language circles around it, we don't like to name it, cross the road to avoid those recently touched by it and shy away from the physical, squeamish fact of it.

Most people want to die at home; most die in hospital. Most want to be with family; often they are alone or with strangers. During the years of John's Campaign we have received hundreds of letters and emails from people whose loved one died in pain, died in fear, died neglected, malnourished, dehydrated, restrained. Died alone. Have we lost our way with dying and with death?

A beloved friend described the death of his wife at too early an age. She was at home, in their bedroom, and by the end was clearly suffering, but hanging on. My friend summoned their two children, who were not yet teenagers, and told them that their mother needed their permission to leave. They sat beside her and each took one of her hands. And they said in turn: 'You can go now, Mum.' And quietly, on the words, she went. She left, and she left them with the gift of herself that they carry still and will always.

Another friend, dying in his forties, tried to get out of his hospital window, as if he could escape death that way.

Sean and I went to see our friend Nick just an hour or so before he died. He knew he was nearly there. The morphine was making him woozy – he thought that the floppy quince blossoms that his wife had put at the end of his bed were ballerinas dancing for him in their pink tutus. He had no religious faith, but he was good-humoured as he lay dying, propped up on the pillow. 'Nearly too late,' he quipped when we came in. We read poems to him (I remember Sean chose Tennyson's 'Now Sleeps the Crimson Petal' and I 'The Sunlight on the Garden' by Louis MacNeice), and then our time was up. 'We've got to go,' I said, and he smiled. 'No, no, it's me who's got to go.' Years later, and I'm still astonished by his wit and grace in the face of his own extinction. Every May, at quince-blossom time, I remember his gallant way of leaving.

Animals perish; only humans die – because we are creatures who are aware of our own mortality. This awareness, which can feel vertiginous, unendurable, is also what gives us selfhood and life shape and meaning. 'Death destroys a man: the idea of Death saves him,' wrote E. M. Forster. It is Henry James's 'distinguished thing', Rochefoucauld's sun that we must not stare at too long lest we go blind with seeing. It makes us and it destroys us.

Dementia has no cure; not yet, anyway. It may take years, it may even take decades, but it is terminal. It comes slowly, creepingly, menacingly. Day by day, week by week, the disease settles in, the sneaky intruder in the house. Doctors, nurses – the whole medical system – are trained to cure people, restoring their patients to the life that was endangered. Hospitals are places of medical intervention, of experts and operating tables and drugs, where death is a failure. In England, more than 50 per cent of deaths take place in hospital, more than 20 per cent in residential and care homes (and only about 8 per cent of people with dementia die in their family home), yet hospitals are not set up to enable people to die well.

But for people who are at the end stages of dementia, death should not be fought against. It's a kindness. Let them go.

Rebecca's mother died towards the end of January 2013, after a period of chaos and distress. The family were reeling under the successive blows the illness had dealt. It had gone on for fourteen years. They had endured more than was possible to endure.

'On the morning of her death,' Rebecca says, 'I had gone home for a short rest. I was walking the dogs and it was a beautiful day. I said the words out loud: "It's all right, Mum. You can go now." I said it. And when the call came, I knew.'

Her face is suffused with tenderness. She pauses for a while, then tells me about her father's death, which happened exactly one year later. He collapsed: 'When I got to the house, I found him being resuscitated by the ambulance crew. I said that this was not what he would want. They said: "Are you asking us to stop?" Oh God. It was awful. I rang my brother and he agreed.' They had learned from experience, and so now she told the paramedics to stop. They stopped. 'They let him go.'

And so it was over, and years have gone by and it's a story that she tells, a tragedy. 'You don't get over it,' she says. 'But you adjust. Of course, they're not here. But they're *here*. In my head. In my heart. I feel their presence and I hear their voice.'

Denis East died in the care home which, by the end, he was no longer trying to escape. His running away was over; his violin playing was over. The Denis East Quartet had ceased to exist – although the trio still visited him and played to him. His daughter, a talented musician herself, came and played the cello, although sometimes he became agitated because he couldn't join in. His grandson played the horn. And Maggie would always make sure he had music on his headphones. He died listening to a Brahms violin sonata. At his funeral, the hymn they sang was 'The Day Thou Gavest, Lord, is Ended'.

The husband of the writer who chose to remain anonymous died peacefully in the home in which he had lived for several months. He had been moved from the dementia unit, where he was distressed by the noise and agitation, to the nursing level, and there had been settled. Then he had a stroke, losing all speech. His wife went to see him every day; they listened to music and she read him *Northanger Abbey*. His son read him poems by Coleridge. 'But it was so constricted a life,' she wrote to me in an email, 'and I couldn't want him to have to bear more. So his slipping away one Sunday night was a grief and a relief.'

Jenni Dutton speaks of her mother's death with joy. 'I was with my mum when she died,' she says. 'It was the most wonderful experience of my life. She was awake and it was the middle of the day. We knew she was dying: she could no longer eat. I watched her, holding her hand, talking and singing to her, telling her how wonderful she was, and how beloved. Very gently, she stopped breathing. And then when someone's dead, they're just *gone*. I've studied my mother's face. That tooth making a bulge in her lip. The light reflecting on the back of her throat as her breath left her body. No pain and no fight – just a glorious amount of gloriousness.'

William Utermohlen died fifteen months after he left home. 'The day he died,' says Pat, 'I was holding a party for my students. The phone rang. They said that Bill was getting ill; there was something wrong with him. I went straightaway. They took him by ambulance to Charing Cross Hospital, and for a while he seemed to be improving. After I'd been there for some time I asked if I had time to go home and have a shower. And, you know, he promptly died. I think he heard me; he must have heard me. I was very relieved; pleased it was over at last for him. He had been so very unhappy. The grieving took place while he was still alive. He died in 2000 when he could no longer draw, and I wasn't sorry when he actually died. I think of the two of us, trotting around the museums of the world together. When I miss him, that's who I'm missing. He was younger than me. He was a quiet man. A very nice, quiet man.'

Death can be a friend. Enough is enough. There has been so much time to prepare and to say goodbye. But when at last they go, we want them back: just a few days longer; just for those words we never spoke; a last farewell. To hold their hand and keep them with us a short while more. Don't go. Please don't go.

My father was one of the lucky few who die at home.

He left us on 9 November 2014. No last words. My mother had said goodnight to him and kissed him. She was in the bathroom cleaning her teeth. His carer was lifting him into a comfortable position on his pillows. He gave a small cough and he died.

We are frail creatures at the last.

The breathing stops and a whole world ends.

Beginnings Again

'Golden lads and girls all must,/As chimney-sweepers, come to dust.'

When people with dementia die their death is often experienced as both loss and release – both for them, who have been dismantled by the illness and have suffered long enough, and for those who loved and cared for them. We say, *They lived beyond their time.* We say, *It was time.* A carer who has spent the last ten years looking after their partner, washing them, feeding them, cleaning up their accidents, weeping over them, recoiling from them, loving them, hating them, bored by the thankless task, trapped by it, exhausted by it, despairing about the lack of reciprocity and their own loss of self, would have to be a saint not to sometimes want them to go, and the long, hard slog to be over. To get a life back.

And then they die and desolation rushes into the spaces carved out by these wretched, unavoidable feelings. Because even though we say that people with dementia are 'gone', are 'husks', are 'not the person they used to be', are the 'walking dead', what we discover when they die is that they were after all still alive. They were after all themselves, although they had lost their self. The difference between my father a few weeks before he died, with his smile that only he ever smiled, and his small chuckle that no one else will give again – the difference between that and the man who I saw dead in the small room at the funeral director's is unquantifiable. People have said to me that there is a spectrum: someone is unequivocally themselves at one end but they gradually slide towards self-loss, so that in a coma, for example, they might be breathing, but they have gone. Nothing remains but the body. A friend of mine had to decide at what point to turn off the machine that was keeping her partner alive: he was in a vegetative state and she had no doubt that it was the only thing to do. But it was a solemn, wrenching decision. To say: this life is over. To say: never more. They will not come again.

And there's the great mystery of life. A person might have nothing left, no memory, no language, no consciousness that they exist in the world. And yet, in this broken body of theirs, some indelible essence of themselves is lodged.

I had been due to go and see my father on the Tuesday, two days after the day on which he died. We knew he didn't have many weeks left, and I had planned which poems I was going to read to him, and what I wanted to say. To thank him. To tell him how well he'd done. To hold his hand, stroke his soft white hair, say goodbye. I wanted to see him one more time before he died – or perhaps it was more that, as soon as he died, I wanted to see him one more time, because although I had thought I was ready for his death, it turned out of course that I wasn't. For so many years – most of my life – I had taken him for granted, a modest, clever, kind, honourable, maverick man who didn't have a mean bone in his body and who cheerfully put his shoulder to life. Just our father. When he died, I stopped taking him for granted. Everything about him became infinitely precious: the way he loved to feed the plain brown birds that came to the bird table in winter; the way he knew how to tie knots and mend china; the way he ate with such deliberation, putting food in small, neat packages on to his fork; the way he took painstaking care over shaving (when I was little, I used to love watching him shave, the rasp of the razor, the line of smooth cheek, just as I used to love watching my mother getting ready to go out, holding loops of beads against her dress, pressing her lipsticked mouth on to a tissue . . .); his absent-mindedness, his eccentric belief in water-divining and the power of dreams; his ancient moss-green jersey; his polished brown shoes; his particular smell . . .

Well, of course, everyone is unique. ('There will be no one like us when we're gone,' writes the dying Oliver Sacks, 'but then there is no one like anyone else ever. When people die, they cannot be replaced. They leave holes that cannot be filled.')

So instead, I came back from a concert and turned on my mobile phone and saw there were several missed calls from my brother. I knew immediately what he wanted to tell me and, sure enough, when I rang him back, he did, in his kind, distressed voice that I know as well as I know any voice in the world. I drove through the small hours and arrived at my parents' house, which was in darkness. I let myself in and went at once to the small room where my father had been lying for the last nine months, and he wasn't there. His body had already been taken away. I stood blinking in the doorway and stared at the narrow, stripped bed and waited in the silence to know what it was I was feeling.

Like when you cut your finger and wait to see blood well up and feel the first throb of pain.

Unreal.

(I have never really cried over my father. I didn't – don't – know where to begin or perhaps, once begun, how I would ever stop. But when I took our anxious, eager old dog to the vet to have her put down, then I cried. She used to come to Sweden with us every summer and she loved to jump into the lake where my father also swam, in his eerie twilight. We would hurl sticks for her and she would launch herself in the air and crash into the water, over and over and over again. I lay on the floor beside her and stroked her and told her we all loved her. I told her that she was going to be always in that lake now, swimming through the water lilies. She thumped her tail gently and then she stopped thumping it. I wept then, because it's easy to weep over a pet: a pure, uncomplicated sorrow. Tears for the dog permitting tears for the man.

And remembering this, another memory comes to me: one of my father's oldest and closest friends died in his forties. I never saw my father shed a tear over it – he wasn't a man who cried easily – but some days later our ancient grey cat died and I found him sitting at his desk, tears sliding unchecked down his face; so very sad, so alone.)

The body dies, is lowered into the ground for its slow absorption back into nature or burnt into ash. But everything that made up that person's inner world – all the love and hope and longing; all the relationships and desires and appetites and curiosities; all the knowledge they built up over the decades; all the memories they had; all their little habits and eccentricities; their intricacy and strangeness and inimitable them-ness; their particular gestures; the way that they smiled; the way the world shaped them and no one else has that shape now or ever will – does this just go?

How can the dead be dead? We talk to them, an impossible conversation, ask their advice, confess our sorrows and desires, seek their approval, have a relationship with them that shifts and changes. We carry them in our hearts. Who are we talking to when we talk to the dead; who are we weeping to when we go to the graveside and pour out our troubles? Who are we loving? For the love is present even when the person is lost, and it reaches into the future even though the future yawns terrifyingly because the person is not in it.

The dead do not die. But they are emphatically dead. They will not come again. The clothes hang in the wardrobe. The chair by the window is empty. The bed is undisturbed.

'To learn to live,' writes Derrida, 'is to learn to live with ghosts, in the upkeep, the conversation, the company or companionship . . . of ghosts.' The ghost is the other, living on in us – because it is only in us that the dead can survive. We have to be haunted. It is very hard to use the past tense.

What is it to mourn? The five stages of grief that Elizabeth Kübler-Ross identifies in her 1969 book *On Death and Dying* (denial, anger, bargaining, depression, acceptance) have for many years been criticized and disputed for their lack of empirical evidence, and for the tidy flatness with which they try to lay a grid over the chaos of grief. Yet the notion of *stages* through which a bereaved person moves retains a powerful grip on us. We want to feel that there is a known way through the bewildering, often disorderly, sometimes brutal mess of emotions; we call it a 'journey', as if there's a map and a compass, steps that should be taken and a place we are trudging towards, even when we know we are lost.

I have a friend whose partner died when he was still young and their child was only four years old. She says that for many months she was quite mad with grief – and she means it literally. She lost her mind over it.

Another talks about how grief *hurts*, physically hurts. In the stomach, in the heart, in the head, in the bones and in the blood. It grabs us, punches at us, takes our breath away, assaults us and wrings us out.

Or another, who speaks of how old she felt for a while – stooped over and slow and befuddled with loss.

Or garrulous, stopping everyone to say over and over again what they have lost; on a loop of time, in perpetual lament.

Or lost, wild, abandoned, scattered. The mind like a drawer of knives.

Useless. Listless. Drab. Tired. Ill: ill with loss.

Strange, unfamiliar; sorrow covers the world like snow does a landscape, making everything that was known strange.

Time passes, a calendar of pain. But death is not just a mark on a headstone. Love is not in the past tense.

A few years ago, as my children were in the process of leaving home, I trained to be a humanist celebrant – conducting funeral services for those who have no faith. Whereas in religious funerals there is a structure and purpose – to consign the dead person to the afterlife, in the hope of being reunited there with them – in humanist ceremonies there is no belief in immortality or hope of ever seeing that person again. How should we say goodbye and not be crushed by the forever-sadness of it?

I met one woman who, in her early sixties, knew that she was close to death and wanted to be part of the funeral arrangements that her stricken family would have to make. She had no belief in the afterlife and yet at one point in our very brief friendship, she said to me: 'When I'm lying in the church in my coffin, I want to know I'm in good hands.' She was graceful, composed, thinking only of the people she was leaving behind who weren't ready to lose her. She was spending her last days writing farewell letters, wrapping presents for her grandchildren, even making sure the freezer was well stocked with her family's favourite meals. She knew her grown-up sons were going to suffer and she was trying to find ways to comfort them from beyond the grave.

Or a son and daughter, in their early twenties, saying goodbye to their magnificent-sounding mother. They were determined to celebrate her in the style in which she had lived, and so they instructed all the mourners to dress to the nines. They wore theatrical clothes, knowingly acting out their grief, and they played joyful music, told funny stories, gave everyone gaudy necklaces to loop around their necks. It was high ritual, kooky, witty and intense.

On another occasion, I helped a mother bury her beloved son. She wrote a poem addressed to him that she read at the funeral, and she spoke of him in a muddle of tenses – past and present and still to come, dead and yet alive and hearing her lines of sorrow. She said that she kept looking out of the window, expecting to see him walking up the garden path. She didn't know what to do with herself or how to get through the days. Every minute dragged at her; every night she waited for the dawn.

Bereavement makes time into a torment. It seems endless and unendurable. We are trapped in it, but the dead person is free, beyond pain at last.

To be human is to feel grief. We do not 'get over' loss (as if it's a barbed-wired fence), nor, like on the bear hunt, do we go round it. I don't even think we go through it, exactly, because that is to assume we come out the other side and are free. It feels more helpful to think of mourning as a gradual taking-into the self of the dead person: once they were external, a beloved object, their own subject; now they are interior, existing in the minds and memories of those they left behind. We lose them – and at the same time we can no longer lose them because they are within us, part of us.

In the past (in Victorian times, for instance, following Queen Victoria's lavish example) there were rules for mourning. These often included social seclusion and mourning clothes that were the outward signs of inward distress. For men, it was easy: a dark suit with black gloves. For women, it was more elaborate: the deep, dull black of a material like unreflective silk or bombazine (very common in novels of the period), trimmed with scratchy crêpe that could be removed after a specified stretch of time ('slighting the mourning'). Jewellery was forbidden, except for jet. There was black material on the door. The clock was sometimes stopped at the time of death. The closing of shutters and pulling-down of blinds – that becomes, in Wilfred Owen's 'Anthem for a Doomed Youth', the soft beauty of 'at each slow dusk a drawing-down of blinds'. The black armbands.

Today, in the Western world at least, we tend to mourn silently and invisibly. Our blinds are not drawn down and our clothes not black (except at some funerals, and even this is getting less common: at many of the services I've conducted mourners are explicitly asked *not* to wear black but bright, celebratory colours). There's often a briskness about the way we deal with death. The number of days a bereaved person is given off work is left to an employer's discretion; most employees have the statutory right to a 'reasonable' amount of unpaid time off under the Employment Rights Act to allow them to deal with unforeseen matters and emergencies involving a dependant. This includes leave to arrange or attend a funeral. (What's 'reasonable' in this time when reason goes sailing out of the window?) The average length of compassionate leave is apparently three to five days. As in the US, where there is no specific provision for bereavement leave, it's largely a matter for employers to decide, and there is no statutory right to be paid. It's as if death is a blip, a glitch – a few days off and we go stoically back to work. We are expected to *get on* with things and *get over* them.

The rituals, which we have now largely lost, publicly recognized the enormity of a death; the recently bereaved were marked out as different. Displaying their status as the mourner, they were distinct in their sorrow, to be treated with sympathy, delicacy and tact. Then, after a set period of time, the deep black gave way to a less inky black; then dark grey, mauve, white. The strict seclusion of the first few months gradually lifted. Mourning turned to half-mourning. Normal life returned slowly, visibly, in stages. The clock was wound up again; time moved forward.

Time stops for those who die, but for their survivors it goes on, ticking and tocking us into the future the dead do not have. For all the agony, the refusal, the dragging of heels and looking back into the underworld, most people let time take them onwards. At the memorial service for the great *Observer* photographer Jane Bown (who I worked alongside for many years, admired and was very fond of), her friend Luke Dodd read a passage from a letter that Samuel Beckett wrote to Barbara Bray in condolence for a recent hard loss. Luke later sent me the text: 'I wish I could find something to comfort you . . . I have so little light and wisdom in me when it comes to such disaster, that I can see nothing for us but the old earth turning onward and time feasting on our suffering along with the rest.' Why is such bleakness a solace? Yet it is: to acknowledge death's harshness and still say that 'somewhere at the heart of the gales of grief (and of love too, I've been told) already they have blown themselves out. I was always grateful for that humiliating consciousness and it was always there huddled, in the innermost place of human frailty and loneliness.' It is the passing of time that he places his faith in: 'Work your head off, sleep at any price and leave the rest to the stream, to carry now away and bring you your other happy days.'

'Surviving – that is the other name of mourning,' writes Derrida. Surviving is a complicated business. Successful mourning is also failed mourning. Grief is an act of memory, of fidelity and of remaining with the person who has died. Recovery is a necessary betrayal and an act of moving forward alone. Many bereaved people feel guilty when they experience moments of returning happiness or realize that for a stretch of time they haven't thought of their loved dead one. The dead become, even briefly, the *forgotten*. And we have to forget, to let the dead gradually sink into our deep memory, where they are not always felt. We would go mad if we did not do this but remained stuck at the first stage of raw, appalled grief (and, of course, people do get stuck and do go mad). The dead are still alive in us, but we do not always remember them because they become part of us, in our fabric. They are forever absent and in the past, and forever present and in our future. This is the work of mourning; painful, time-consuming, solemn, crucial work. To gather the dead to ourselves; to recognize our own mortality.

Death is never a slight thing, however peaceful a passing is, however minute the distance crossed. Just a breath away, then like a feather being blown with a single puff and a whole world has disappeared.

And yet death can also restore a person, especially when that person had been un-made by dementia. Once they die, they are no longer only old and frail and ill, they are no longer only confused and forgetful, no longer a wrecked body and a failing mind, no longer not themselves. Because they have gone from us, they can come back to us and be all the selves they have ever been. Young, old, everything in between. Robust, vulnerable, everything in between. And often we fall head over heels in love with all these selves and we understand how they contained multitudes. (How we all contain multitudes.)

This is what good funerals can bring: the sense of a whole self being recollected again, restored and redeemed. Time, which is so tyrannical, releases its chronological grip. I was the celebrant for the funeral of a friend's husband, who had lived with and died of Lewy body dementia. His illness and his last months were not denied during the service, which was largely written by his family, but were touched on then laid aside to make way for the rest of his long and good life: a man who had loved the sea and fishing, who had loved cooking, eating, laughing, joking; who had loved his children, who had loved his wife.

We talk of 'funeral directors' now, as though a funeral were a corporate event. They used to be called undertakers – which is what the American poet Thomas Lynch still calls himself, for he loves the way the word collects up many meanings (the taking under ground, the task, the pledge). 'From something done with the dead, to something done for the living, to something done by the living – every one of us.' He believes that 'undertakings are the things that we do to vest the lives we lead against the cold, the meaningless, the void, the noisome blather and the blinding dark. It is the voice we give to wonderment, to pain, to love and desire, anger and outrage; the words that we shape into song and prayer.' And towards the end of *The Undertaking: Life Studies from the Dismal Trade*, he adds this urgent advice: 'Whatever's there to feel, feel it – the riddance, the relief, the fright and freedom, the fear of forgetting, the dull ache of your own mortality . . . The only way round these things is through them.'

We four siblings arranged and conducted my father's funeral. His grandchildren, each grandson wearing one of his ties, carried the wicker coffin that they had decorated with flowers that morning, and they stood together at the front of the hall to one by one share a particular memory they had of their grandfather. Two of his old friends told stories about him, funny and affectionate. We all sang the hymn that had been sung at my parents' wedding, 'Dear Lord and Father of Mankind'. And we four told his life together and remembered all the things he had most loved, that we had most loved in him. We each read a poem. My eldest sister (who shares with him a passionate attachment to the natural world) read Gerald Manley Hopkins's 'Pied Beauty'. My brother read Henry Reed's Second World War poem 'Naming of Parts' – one of my father's all-time favourites, though none of us ever quite knew why. My sister, who loves sailing, as did he, read John Masefield's 'Sea Fever'. And I read Thomas Hardy's 'Afterwards', the poet's rueful elegy to himself as 'a man who used to notice such things':

> When the Present has latched its postern behind my
>   tremulous stay,
> And the May month flaps its glad green leaves
>   like wings,
> Delicate-filmed as new-spun silk, will the
>   neighbours say,
> 'He was a man who used to notice such things'?

That poem puts the dead person beautifully in the past and shuts the gate behind him, but there was a sense during his funeral that our father was present: in the room, in our minds, our memories, our hearts. And he wasn't demented any more, he wasn't helpless and ashamed and scared and lost. He was smiling, strong, full of health. He was happy again. This was good grief, rich and full and clear, very different from the harrowing wretchedness of the past year.

Siegfried Sassoon once wrote to a bereaved friend, 'You are rich in all you have lost.' We are rich in all that we lose. The more we have, the more we lose; and the more we lose, the richer we are. Grief is a torment and a blessing.

So the old man in *Alive Inside* will swing around the lamp posts once more, taking his daughter to school.

So the old woman I saw lying slack in a hospital bed will also be the young woman in the photograph, standing hand in hand with her beau on a seashore, smiling.

So Denis East can pick up his violin again and play Mendelssohn and Bach and Beethoven's Opus 131.

And Rebecca Myers's mother can dance with her adoring husband again, and Rebecca can lay her head on her mother's shoulder and tell all her troubles.

And Jenni Dutton's mother can be knitted up, her face emerging from the skein of loose threads.

And Theresa Clarke can be Teasie, and the boys all want her to come and play football; and she will be at peace in her ashram, and at the source of the Ganges, where she always dreamed of going; and her mother can tell her she has the heart of a lion.

And Tommy Dunne will see his Joyce and think that the sun rises when she does.

And William Utermohlen can wander around the museums and art galleries of the world with the woman he loves, staring at paintings that he stores inside his head. And he can pick up his brush again. The scribbled face on a flat white background, the wild empty eyes and the nose like a beak of a bird, will transform. The anxious sadness will ebb away. Colours will seep back, and perspectives; walls will straighten and the vertigo of distress be banished. The lonely figure on the edge of a group, looking on, will sit at the table again, among the conversation and the laughter.

And my father can listen to the dawn chorus again. He can walk around his garden, watering the tomatoes in the greenhouse, pruning the roses and feeding the small brown songbirds. He can tie knots deftly and mend china so you can't tell it was ever broken. Drive a car, read a map, sail a boat, solve a crossword clue, paint a watercolour landscape, fork the compost, tease his grandchildren, stare intently at an insect on a leaf, drink a glass of good red wine, dance the foxtrot again and the waltz, sing carols and folk songs, laugh with friends, light bonfires and look at stars, hold my mother's hand, set going the grandfather clock that stands in the hall and hear the steady tick of time passing, close the curtains and turn off the lights, blow out the candles, walk up the stairs and climb into bed, say goodnight and close his eyes, dream his dreams.

So many selves that death releases back into the world; ghosts that do not haunt us but accompany us, or we accompany them, as we go towards our own endless night.

The bright day is done. We all come to darkness.

To reach the end. To end with love.

Notes on Sources

p. vii 'Abyss has no Biographer': from Emily Dickinson's letters ('To attempt to speak of what has been, would be impossible. Abyss has no Biographer'), quoted by Lyndall Gordon in *Lives Like Loaded Guns: Emily Dickinson and Her Family's Feuds*, p. 7

Beginnings

p. i 'Oh the mind, mind has mountains . . .': from one of Gerard Manley Hopkins's great Sonnets of Desolation, 'No Worst', in *Poems and Prose* (London: Everyman's Library, 1995):

> O the mind, mind has mountains; cliffs of fall
> Frightful, sheer, no-man-fathomed. Hold them cheap
> May who ne'er hung there . . .

p. 4 'disease of the century': from the Introduction to *Dementia and Ageing: Ethics, Values and Policy Choices*, ed. Robert H. Binstock, Stephen G. Post and Peter J. Whitehouse, p. ix

p. 4 'the story of suffering': from 'Seeing and Knowing Dementia', by David H. Smith, in *Dementia and Ageing: Ethics, Values and Policy Choices*, p. 49

p. 4 'Dementia is profoundly disrespectful of patients, carers, health systems, social care . . . it doesn't fit into the structures we've created': from my interview with Professor Sube Banerjee, Professor of Dementia and Associate Dean at Brighton and Sussex Medical School

p. 7 The world 'is given to us in common': from an interview with Judith Butler in the *Other Journal*, issue 27, 26 June 2017

p. 9 Mary Warnock made her remark in the Church of Scotland's *Life and Work* magazine, as reported in, for example, *Telegraph*, 18 September 2008

p. 10 'the endurance of the soul': from Atul Gawande's *Being Mortal*, p. 231

p. 11 Dante's image of a boat lowering its sails ('to furl our sail and take our rigging in'): from *The Divine Comedy, Inferno*, Canto 27, ll. 79–81

p. 12 Sally Magnusson uses the image of a boat going into the mist in her memoir, *Where Memories Go: Why Dementia Changes Everything*, p. 91

p. 12 'a sailing vessel that is becalmed . . .': from *Out of Mind* by J. Bernlef, p. 54

p. 12 Erwin Mortier's desolating and beautiful *Stammered Songbook* is made of metaphors and is in part about the impossibility of language to capture its own disintegration. For the metaphors quoted here, see pp. 10, 11, 19, 50, 65, 107 . . .

p. 14 'To be human is to have a voice': the ethicist Carol Gilligan eloquently articulates the central meaning of the human voice in her important book, *In a Different Voice: Psychological Theory and Women's Development*

p. 15 'I write partly to make a confession': Oliver Sacks made this remark in an interview with Drouwe Draaisma, Professor of the History of Psychology at the University of Groningen, in the Netherlands. It is quoted in Draaisma's *The Nostalgia Factory: Memory, Time and Ageing*, p. 112

p. 15 To write is to ask for forgiveness: the French philosopher Jacques Derrida wrote extensively (and influentially) about death, mourning and forgiveness. Whereas Freud viewed mourning as normalizing work, a journey through grief to relinquishment and consolation, for Derrida it is a great, always unfinished work in which we continue to talk to the dead. See, for example, his *Adieu to Emmanuel Levinas*, or Nicholas Royle's discussion in *In Memory of Jacques Derrida*

1. *Facing Up*

p. 17 'I am! yet what I am none cares or knows': 'I Am!' by John Clare, from *John Clare*

p. 27 The acronym 'GOMERs' was first coined by the pseudonymous American doctor Samuel Shen in his 1978 novel *House of God*

pp. 27–8 For the story about the ninety-five-year-old man who tried to kill his wife, see, for example, the *Guardian*, 25 April 2017

p. 28 Dementia 'seriously jeopardizes the faculties we ordinarily define as uniquely human . . .': from Robert N. Butler's Foreword to *Dementia and Ageing: Ethics, Values and Policy Choices*, ed. Robert H. Binstock, Stephen G. Post and Peter J. Whitehouse

p. 28 'What it is that dementia takes away? . . .': from Andrea Gillies's *Keeper*, p. 11

2. *Getting Older*

p. 29 'Oldness has come . . . the heart is forgetful': from an Ancient Egyptian scroll, quoted by Carmelo Aquilino and Julian C. Hughes in their essay, 'The Return of the Living Dead, in *Dementia: Mind, Meaning and the Person*, ed. Julian C. Hughes, Stephen J. Louw and Stephen R. Sabat, p. 143

p. 29 'you will be old for longer than you were ever young': from Drouwe Draaisma's *The Nostalgia Factory: Memory, Time and Ageing*, p. 6

p. 29 The statistics on population ageing are taken from the UN Report, 'World Population Ageing 2015', the UN Department of Economic and Social Affairs, Population Division New York

p. 32 'them' not 'us': see Simone de Beauvoir's *Old Age*

p. 33 'temporal vertigo': from Lynne Segal's *Out of Time: The Pleasures and Perils of Ageing*, p. 4

p. 36 'the contradiction between inner and outer of a different order to anything we have previously faced': from Helen Small's *The Long Life*, p. 12

p. 36 Montaigne's 'special favour' and 'privilege': quoted by Helen Small in *The Long Life*, p. 2

p. 37 'Please, *please*, don't talk to me about old age so much . . . You are giving me the creeps! . . .': from *Words in Air: The Complete Correspondence between Elizabeth Bishop and Robert Lowell*, p. 779. Elizabeth Bishop was only sixty-three when she wrote this, and Lowell fifty-eight!

p. 37 'alacrity': quoted by Helen Small in *The Long Life*, p. 2

p. 37 'abundance': see Annie Dillard's book of that name

p. 37 'touch the ceiling': from *Words in Air: The Complete Correspondence between Elizabeth Bishop and Robert Lowell*, p. 681

p. 37 'The story of ageing is the story of our parts . . .': from Atul Gawande's *Being Mortal*, p. 29

p. 38 'something is not quite right': from Drouwe Draaisma's *The Nostalgia Factory: Memory, Time and Ageing*, p. 1

p. 38 Tad Friend's article, 'Silicon Valley's Quest to Live Forever' appeared in the *New Yorker* issue of 3 April 2017

pp. 38–40 Ezekiel Emanuel wrote about his decision to receive only palliative treatment beyond the age of seventy-five in the *Atlantic* in October 2014

p. 40 'The body ages. The body is preparing to die . . .': from John Berger's *And our faces, my heart, brief as photos*, p. 36

3. The Brain, the Mind and the Self

p. 43 'the marvel of consciousness . . .': Vladimir Nabokov, quoted in Brian Boyd's *Vladimir Nabokov: The Russian Years*, p. 11

p. 48 Drouwe Draaisma gives the figure of 256 in *The Nostalgia Factory: Memory, Time and Ageing*, p. 33

p. 51 'transient electrochemical dance, made of myriad bits of information': from Henry Marsh's *Admissions*, p. 267

p. 55 For the full story of the life and death of Sandy Bem, see the long piece in the *New York Times*, 15 May 2015

p. 62 Peter Singer's list of indicators for personhood, as given in Stephen G. Post's *The Moral Challenge of Alzheimer's Disease*, p. 15

p. 62 'Neither *cogito* (I think) nor *ergo* (therefore) but *sum*: I am': ibid., p. 3

p. 62 'the socially outcast, the unwanted, the marginalized and the oppressed': ibid.

4. Memory and Forgetting

p. 64 'All this goes on inside me, in the vast cloisters of my memory . . .': from St Augustine's *Confessions*, p. 215

p. 64 'Life without memory is no life at all': from Luis Buñuel's autobiography, *My Last Breath*, pp. 4–5. At the end of her life, Buñuel's mother had no memory left, and the fuller extract reads: 'to begin to lose your memory, if only in bits and pieces, [is] to realize that memory is what makes our lives. Life without memory is no life at all . . . our memory is our coherence, our reason, our feeling, even our action. Without it, we are nothing.'

p. 65 'the world glides through you without leaving a trace': from J. Bernlef's *Out of Mind*, p. 41

p. 66 The 'permastore' of long-term memory: from Drouwe Draaisma's *The Nostalgia Factory: Memory, Time and Ageing*, p. x

p. 68 For the many metaphors of storage, see Charles Fernyhough's *Pieces of Light: The New Science of Memory*, p. 6

p. 68 'If only this could be your memory . . .': from Drouwe Draaisma's *Forgetting: Myths, Perils and Compensations*, p. 1

p. 68 Memory as an 'an activity, not a vault . . . a process not a place' and 'like an orchestra': from Andrea Gillies's *Keeper*, p. 228

p. 69 memory is 'a seamstress, a capricious one at that . . .': from Virginia Woolf's *Orlando*, p. 49

p. 69 'there are no "read only" files': from Drouwe Draaisma's *Forgetting: Myths, Perils and Compensations*, p. 8

p. 69 forgetting as the 'minus sign . . .', and the lack of a verbal equivalent of memory: ibid, p. 1

p. 69 For an account of HSAM, see the long article in the *Guardian*, 8 February 2017

p. 69 the 'garbage heap' of memory, from 'Funes the Memorious,' in *The Total Library: Non-fictions, 1922–1986*, by Jorge Luis Borges, p. 96

p. 76 Patrice Polini's psychoanalytic analysis of Utermohlen's art is found in his essay 'Conveying the Experience of Alzheimer's Disease through Art: The Later Paintings of William Utermohlen', from *Looking into Later Life*, ed. Rachel Davenhill, pp. 298–318

5. The Diagnosis

p. 83 'We have heard the chimes at midnight': from *Henry IV*, Part 2

p. 91 Michael Kinsley wrote his defence of denial in *Time Magazine*, 9 December 2004

p. 99 'courage to be': from Stephen G. Post's *The Moral Challenge of Alzheimer's Disease*, p. 1

6. Shame

p. 100 'Pray, do not meck me . . .': from *King Lear*, Act IV, Scene vii

p. 106 'crucial part of self-respect is respect in the eyes of others . . .': from 'A Critical View of Ethical Dilemmas' by Harry Moody, in *Dementia and Ageing: Ethics, Values and Policy Choices*, ed. Robert H. Binstock, Stephen G. Post and Peter J. Whitehouse, p. 90

p. 106 'sound in oneself of the voice of judgement': from Bernard Williams's *Shame and Necessity*, p. 89

p. 107 'that of being seen, inappropriately . . .': ibid., p. 78

p. 107 'The other sees all of me, and all through me . . .': ibid., p. 89

p. 107 For an exploration of the connection between shame and death, see Carl Schneider's *Shame, Exposure and Privacy*

p. 107 'The contradiction between inner and outer . . .': from Helen Small's *The Long Life*, p. 12

7. The Carers

p. 114 'How far that little candle throws his beam': from *The Merchant of Venice*, Act V, Scene 1

p. 114 The statistics on carers are taken from Carers UK, 'Facts about Carers 2015'; Alzheimer's Research UK's Dementia Statistics Hub, 'Impact on Carers', 2015; and the Family Care Giver Alliance, 'Caregiver Statistics: Demographics,' 2016

p. 117 Frédéric Compain's short and beautiful film is called *William Utermohlen: Vision intérieure de la maladie d'Alzheimer*

p. 118 'She has possessed me and I am diminished': from Andrea Gillies's *Keeper*, p. 237

p. 119 Sally Gadow is quoted by Richard J. Martin and Stephen G. Post in 'Human Dignity, Dementia and the Basis of Caregiving', from *Dementia and Ageing: Ethics, Values, and Policy Choices*, ed. Robert H. Binstock, Stephen G. Post and Peter J. Whitehouse, p. 57

p. 121 This account of Jane English's question 'What do children owe their parents?' is taken from 'Human Dignity, Dementia and the Basis of Caregiving' by Richard J. Martin and Stephen G. Post, in *Dementia and Ageing: Ethics, Values and Policy Choices*, ed. Robert H. Binstock, Stephen G. Post and Peter J. Whitehouse, p. 60

p. 121 filial obligation can serve as a 'maleficent ideological warrant for the destruction of daughters': ibid., p. 61

8. *Connecting through the Arts*

p. 143 'And hand in hand, on the edge of the sand . . .': 'The Owl and the Pussycat' by Edward Lear, in *The Complete Nonsense of Edward Lear*

9. *Home*

p. 154 'You can go home again . . .': from Ursula Le Guin's *The Dispossessed*, p. 48

pp. 157, 159 Home is 'at the heart of the real'; to be 'shelterless . . . undoing the very meaning of the world . . .': Mircea Eliade, quoted by John Berger in *And our faces, my heart, brief as photos*, pp. 55–6

p. 159 'the raw material of repetitions turned into a shelter', memory as the 'mortar that binds the improvised home together', 'return to where distance did not yet count': ibid., p. 64

p. 159 'a precise and uncomplicated conviction the world was available to me . . .': from Hisam Matar's *The Return: Fathers, Sons and the Land in Between*, p. 126

p. 161 These statistics about abuse are taken from the *Nursing Home Abuse Guide*

p. 161 For the statistics of elderly abuse by carers in the UK see, for example, the *Telegraph*, 28 February 2017, or the *Guardian*, 2 March 2017

p. 162 'We end up with institutions that address any number of societal goals . . .': from Atul Gawande's *Being Mortal*, p. 77

p. 172 'we shall not cease from exploration . . .' T. S. Eliot's *Four Quartets*, 'Little Gidding', Part V

p. 172 'searing' homesickness for the site of 'psychic security', 'abandonment and dread': from 'Only Connect' by Margot Waddell, in *Looking into Later Life: A Psychoanalytic Approach to Depression and Dementia in Old Age*, ed. Rachel Davenhill, pp. 194–5

p. 172 At death, men apparently long for their mother; women for the time when they were the mothers of young children: from Drouwe Draaisma's *The Nostalgia Factory: Memory, Time and Ageing*

10. *The Later Stages*

p. 175 'I'm all these words, all these strangers . . .': *The Unnameable* by Samuel Beckett, p. 104

pp. 177–8 Atul Gawande's article was in the issue of 30 March 2009

12. *At the End*

p. 194 'We possess art lest we perish of the truth': fragment 822, Book 3 of Nietzsche's *Will to Power*

p. 198 'To have a voice is to be human . . .': from Carol Gilligan's *In a Different Voice: Psychological Theory and Women's Development*, p. xvi

p. 199 'they are ignorant of self . . .': from Helen Small's discussion of Ronald Dworkin in *The Long Life*, p. 130

p. 199 'I–Thou'. 'Speech does not reside in man . . .': from 'Seeing Whole', the opening essay by Julian C. Hughes, Stephen J. Louw and Steven R. Sabat, in *Dementia: Mind, Meaning and the Person*, p. 26

p. 200 'ruins of grammar . . .' from 'The Hard Words'; 'forever in my mouth/ and forgetting' from 'Left Brain'; 'dirty taste of gone' from 'Right Brain': all from Sarah Hesketh's *The Hard Word Box*

p. 200 This account of Swift's last years and of his death comes from John Gray's article in the *New Statesman*, 14 November 2016

p. 201 To 'fix an image of the self', and 'calling forth his double', from Patrice Polini's essay in Rachel Davenhill's *Looking into Later Life*

13. *Saying Goodbye*

p. 207 'What is loss? Loss is a sleeping giant': from Marion Coutts's *Iceberg*, p. 73

14. *Death*

p. 214 'Death twitches. "Live," he says. "I am coming." ': Virgil, quoted by Christine Overall in *Ageing, Death and Human Longevity*, p. 1

p. 216 Animals do not die, only perish: for a development of this idea, see p. 50 of 'Ageing and Human Nature' by Michael Bavidge, in *Dementia: Mind, Meaning and the Person*, ed. Julian C. Hughes, Stephen J. Louw and Steven R. Sabat: 'only creatures who are self-consciously aware of themselves as individuals can die – and only creature who are aware of their own deaths develop notions of themselves as individuals'

p. 216 'Death destroys a man: the idea of Death saves him': from E. M. Forster's *Howards End*, chapter 27

p. 216 'distinguished thing': Henry James cited by Louis Menand in the *New Yorker*, 21 July 2016

p. 216 These figures for where people die are taken from Public Health England's official statistics, published in 2018

Beginnings Again

p. 220 'Golden lads and girls all must,/As chimney sweepers, come to dust': from *Cymbeline*, Act IV, Scene 2

p. 221 'There will be no one like us when we're gone . . .': from Oliver Sacks's *Gratitude*, p. 19

p. 224 'To learn to live, is to learn to live with ghosts . . .': from Nicholas Royle's *In Memory of Jacques Derrida*, p. 71

p. 227 I am paraphrasing a piece in the *Guardian*, 10 January 2014, about bereavement leave

p. 228 'I wish I could find something to comfort you . . .': Samuel Beckett wrote these words to Barbara Bray on 10 March 1958

p. 229 'Surviving – that is the other name for mourning': from Jacques Derrida's *The Work of Mourning*, p. 1

p. 230 'From something done with the dead . . .': from *The Undertaking* by Thomas Lynch, p. xviii

p. 230 'Undertakings are the things that we do . . .': ibid., p. xix

Bibliography

Agronin, Marc E. *How We Age* (Cambridge, Mass.; Da Capo Press, 2011)

Andrews, June. *Dementia: The One-stop Guide* (London: Profile Books, 2015)

Ariès, Philippe. *Western Attitudes towards Death* (London: Marion Boyars, 1976)

de Beauvoir, Simone. *Old Age*, trans. Patrick O'Brian (London: Penguin, 1977)

Beckett, Samuel. *The Unnameable* (London: Faber and Faber, 2010)

Berger, John. *Here is Where We Meet* (London: Bloomsbury, 2005)

— *Selected Essays*, ed. Geoff Dyer (London: Bloomsbury, 2001)

—*And our faces, my heart, brief as photos* (New York: Random House, 1984)

Bernlef, J. *Out of Mind*, trans. Adrienne Dixon (London: Faber and Faber, 1980)

—*Eclipse*, trans. Paul Vincent (London: Faber and Faber, 1996)

Binstock, Robert H., Post, Stephen G., Whitehouse, Peter J. (eds.). *Dementia and Ageing: Ethics, Values and Policy Choices* (London: Johns Hopkins University Press, 1992)

Bishop, Elizabeth and Lowell, Robert. *Words in Air: The Complete Correspondence between Elizabeth Bishop and Robert Lowell*, ed. Thomas Travisano and Saskia Hamilton (London: Faber and Faber, 2008)

Borges, Jorge Luis. *The Total Library: Non-fictions 1922–1986*, trans. Esther Allen (London: Penguin, 2001)

—*Fictions*, trans. Andrew Hurley (London: Penguin, 1998)

Bibliography

Boyd, Brian. *Vladimir Nabokov: The Russian Years* (London: Vintage, 1990)

Buñuel, Luis. *My Last Breath*, trans. Abigail Israel (London: Fontana, 1985)

Burdick, Alan. *Why Time Flies: A Mostly Scientific Investigation* (London: Simon and Schuster, 2017)

Butler, Judith. Interview in the *Other Journal*, 27: Identity Issue (Seattle: 27 June 2017)

Clare, John. *John Clare*, ed. Paul Farley (London: Faber and Faber, 2016)

Compain, Frédéric. *William Utermohlen: Vision intérieure de la maladie d'Alzheimer* (Paris: Arts Editions, 2009)

Corkin, Suzanne. *Permanent Present Tense: The Man with No Memory, and What He Taught the World* (London: Penguin, 2013)

Coutts, Marion. *The Iceberg* (Atlantic Books, 2014)

Dante Alighieri. *The Divine Comedy: Inferno*, trans. Robin Kirkpatrick (London: Penguin, 2006)

Dartington, Tim. *Managing Vulnerability* (London: Karnac Books, 2010)

Davenhill, Rachel (ed). *Looking into Later Life: A Psychoanalytic Approach to Depression and Dementia in Old Age* (London: Karnac Books, 2007)

Derrida, Jacques. *The Work of Mourning*, ed. Pascale-Anne Brault and Michael Naas (Chicago: University of Chicago Press: 2017)

—*Adieu to Emmanuel Levinas* (Stanford: Stanford University Press, 1997)

Dillard, Annie. *The Abundance* (Edinburgh: Canongate Books, 2017)

Diski, Jenny. *In Gratitude* (London: Bloomsbury, 2016)

Dollimore, Jonathan. *Death, Desire and Loss in Western Culture* (London: Allen Lane, 1998)

Draaisma, Drouwe. *The Nostalgia Factory: Memory, Time and Ageing*, trans. Liz Waters (London: Yale University Press, 2013)

—*Forgetting: Myths, Perils and Compensations*, trans. Liz Waters (Yale: Yale University Press, 2004)

Eliot, T. S. *The Complete Poems and Plays* (London: Faber and Faber, 1975)

Fernyhough, Charles. *Pieces of Light: The New Science of Memory* (London: Profile Books, 2013)

Forster, E. M. *Howards End* (London: Penguin, 2000)

Francis, Gavin. *Adventures in Human Being* (London: Profile Books, 2015)

Gawande, Atul. *Being Mortal* (London: Profile Books, 2015)

Gillies, Andrea. *Keeper* (London: Short Books, 2009)

Gilligan, Carol. *In a Different Voice: Psychological Theory and Women's Development* (Cambridge, Mass.:, Harvard University Press, 2003)

Gogol, Nikolai. *Dead Souls*, trans. David Magarshak (London: Penguin, 1961)

Gordon, Lyndall. *Lives Like Loaded Guns: Emily Dickinson and Her Family's Feuds* (London: Virago, 2011)

Hardy, Thomas. *Collected Poems*, ed. Samuel Hynes (Oxford: Oxford University Press, 1984)

Healey, Elizabeth. *Elizabeth is Missing* (London: Viking, 2014)

Hesketh, Sarah. *The Hard Word Box* (London: Penned in the Margins, 2014)

Hopkins, Gerard Manley. *Poems and Prose* (London: Everyman's Library, 1995)

Hughes, Julian C., Louw, Stephen J., Sabat, Steven R. *Dementia: Mind, Meaning and the Person* (Oxford: Oxford University Press, 2016)

Ishiguro, Kazuo. *The Unconsoled* (London: Faber and Faber, 1995)

James, Jo, et al. *Excellent Dementia Care in Hospitals* (London: Jessica Kingsley, 2017)

James, William. *The Principles of Psychology*, vol. 1 (London: Forgotten Books, 2017)

Bibliography

Jones, Julia. *Beloved Old Age and What To Do about It* (Essex: Golden Duck, 2016)

Kalanith, Paul. *When Breath Becomes Air* (London: Bodley Head, 2016)

Larkin, Philip: *Collected Poems* (London: Faber and Faber, 1988)

Lear, Edward. *The Complete Nonsense of Edward Lear* (London: Faber and Faber, 2015)

Le Guin, Ursula. *The Dispossessed* (New York: HarperCollins, 1974)

Luria, A. R. *The Man with the Shattered World* (London: Penguin, 1972)

Lynch, Thomas. *Bodies in Motion and at Rest: On Metaphor and Mortality* (London: W. W. Norton, 2000)

—*The Undertaking: Life Studies from the Dismal Trade* (London: Vintage, 1998)

Magnusson, Sally. *Where Memories Go: Why Dementia Changes Everything* (London: John Murray, 2014)

Malouf, David. *An Imaginary Life* (London: Vintage, 1999)

Marsh, Henry. *Admissions: A Life in Brain Surgery* (London: Weidenfeld and Nicolson, 2017)

—*Do No Harm: Stories of Life, Death and Brain Surgery* (London: Phoenix, 2014)

Matar, Hisham. *The Return: Fathers, Sons and the Land in Between* (London: Viking, 2016)

Mayeroff, Milton. *On Caring* (New York: HarperCollins, 1971)

Mortier, Erwin. *Stammered Songbook*, trans. Paul Vincent (London: Pushkin Press, 2015)

Nietzsche, Friedrich. *The Will to Power*, trans. Walter Kaufmann and R. J. Holingdale (New York: Vintage, 1968)

Nuland, Sherwin. *How We Die* (Chatto and Windus, 1994)

Oppen, George. *New Collected Poems* (Manchester: Carcanet Press, 2003)

O'Mahony, Seamus. *The Way We Die Now* (London: Head of Zeus, 2016)

Overall, Christine. *Ageing, Death and Human Longevity* (London: University of California Press, 2003)

Post, Stephen G. *The Moral Challenge of Alzheimer's Disease* (Baltimore: Johns Hopkins University Press, 1995)

Roiphe, Kate. *The Violet Hour: Great Writers at the End* (London: Virago, 2016)

Royle, Nicholas. *In Memory of Jacques Derrida* (Edinburgh: Edinburgh University Press, 2009)

Sacks, Oliver. *Gratitude* (London: Picador, 2015)

—*The Man Who Mistook His Wife for a Hat* (London: Picador, 1986)

St Augustine. *Confessions*, trans. R. S. Pine-Coffin (London: Penguin, 1961)

Samuel, Julia. *Grief Works* (London: Penguin Random House, 2017)

Schneider, Carl. *Shame, Exposure and Privacy* (London: W. W. Norton, 1992)

Segal, Lynne. *Out of Time: The Pleasures and Perils of Ageing* (London: Verso, 2015)

Shem, Samuel. *Black Swan* (London: Transworld, 1998)

Shenk, David. *The Forgetting: Alzheimer's: Portrait of an Epidemic* (New York: Anchor Books, 2001)

Shorthouse, Tracey. *I Am Still Me* (Bloomington, IL: Author House, 2017)

Singer, Peter. *Rethinking Life and Death* (Oxford: Oxford University Press, 1994)

Small, Helen. *The Long Life* (Oxford: Oxford University Press, 2007)

Swaffer, Kate. *What the Hell Happened to My Brain: Living beyond Dementia* (London: Jessica Kingsley, 2016)

Swaffer, Kate and Low, Lee-Fay. *Diagnosed with Alzheimer's or Another Dementia* (London: New Holland Publishers, 2016)

Tallis, Raymond. *The Black Mirror: Fragments of an Obituary for Life* (London: Atlantic Books, 2015)

Taylor, Cory. *Dying: A Memoir* (Edinburgh: Canongate Books, 2016)

Bibliography

Taylor, Richard. *Alzheimer's from the Inside Out* (Baltimore: Health Professions Press, 2004)

Thomas, Matthew. *We are Not Ourselves* (London: Fourth Estate, 2015)

Whitman, Lucy (ed.). *Telling Tales about Dementia: Experiences of Caring* (London: Jessica Kingsley, 2010)

Williams, Bernard. *Shame and Necessity* (London: University of California Press, 1993)

Woolf, Virginia. *Orlando* (London: Vintage Classics, 2016)

Wordsworth, William. *The Oxford Authors*, ed. Stephen Gill (Oxford: Oxford University Press, 1984)

Zeizel, John. *I am Still Here* (London: Piatkus, 2011)

Acknowledgements

I am indebted to more people than I can ever list here; I never even knew the names of some of them. Since the founding of John's Campaign, I have met a great number of wonderful men and women up and down the country who have supported, encouraged, advised, helped and joined us in the fight to make care in hospitals more transparent and compassionate. I will always remember their kindness.

I owe a debt of gratitude to those people I talked to for the book, the nurses and doctors and health professionals, the social workers and psychotherapists and artists, who so generously gave me their time and shared their knowledge; the people who work in care homes and welcomed me in; the friends who let me explore my thoughts in safety: Felicity Allen, Claire Armitstead, Andrew Balfour, Sube Banerjee, Philippa Black, Alistair Burns, Andrew Cooper, Alex Coulter, Seb Crutch, Jane Cummings, Tim Dartington, April Dobson and the staff at Abbeyfield, Steve Gentleman, Lucy Gilby, Gil Graystone, Rowan Harwood, Sarah Hesketh, Jo James, Liz Jones and the staff at MHA, Kate Kellaway, Claire Kent, Jules Knight, James Macdonald, Michael Morris, John Naughton, Jane O'Grady, David Oliver, Aishlene O'Neill, Maria Parsons, Josh Pettit, Hilary Prior, Martin Rossor, Raymond Tallis, Sophia Tickell, Nick Timmins, Carol Tolpolski, Claudia Wald. Their thoughts and their knowledge were invaluable – and all mistakes are mine alone.

My special thanks go to those people who talked to me about

their personal and often very painful experience of dementia. I am bowled over by the generosity, honesty and courage of Gillian Beer, Andy and Claire Bell, Jan Bell, Pam Bell, Theresa Clarke, Joyce Dunne, Tommy Dunne, Jenni Dutton, Maggie East, Mary Jacobus, Disie Johnson, Rebecca Myers, Pauline Teerehorst, Patricia Utermohlen and Gerard de Vries.

I am profoundly grateful to the *Observer* newspaper, without which John's Campaign would never have existed, and without which this book could never have been written. They gave me a platform and a voice. In particular, I want to thank Jane Ferguson, Ursula Kenny, John Mulholland, Lisa O'Kelly, Stephen Pritchard, Paul Webster and Rob Yates for their generous help and steadfast support over all these years.

Julia Jones has been my unswerving friend through good times and bad. My thanks and admiration and love go to her, and to Francis and Bertie Wheen.

A great editor is a great gift. Helen Conford has encouraged me, challenged me, unsettled me, helped me more than I can say. Margaret Stead was always clear, scrupulous, kind and invaluable. Ginny Smith in the US was a great support and gave me the confidence I needed. Thank you.

What Dementia Teaches Us about Love would never have been written without my wonderful, clever, kind agent, Sarah Ballard. From the first idea to the final word, she has been my guide and my safe place. Thanks also go to Eli Keren for his help and patience, to fabulous Sam Edenborough and Nicki Kennedy for their support and faith in me, and to Joy Harris in the US, whose steadfast commitment has meant a great deal.

The book begins in Sweden. Many thanks to the great tribe of Sean's relatives who always welcomed my parents to the crayfish parties, tango lessons and summer celebrations there.

Edgar, Anna, Hadley and Molly (and Phoebe and Tom) lift

me up, keep me going, and make me grateful and happy, every day. And to Sean, my first reader, my coffee-maker and wine-pourer, my fellow traveller, my unconditional without-whom: thank you.

Above all, I am forever grateful to my mother, Patricia Gerrard, my brother Tim Gerrard, my sisters Jackie Gerrard-Reis and Katie Jackson: the best, the most generous-hearted family anyone could have.

And to my father – well, words fail me. Goodbye.

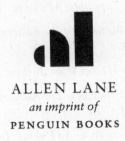

ALLEN LANE

an imprint of

PENGUIN BOOKS

Also Published

Stuart Russell, *Human Compatible: AI and the Problem of Control*

Serhii Plokhy, *Forgotten Bastards of the Eastern Front: An Untold Story of World War II*

Dominic Sandbrook, *Who Dares Wins: Britain, 1979-1982*

Charles Moore, *Margaret Thatcher: The Authorized Biography, Volume Three: Herself Alone*

Thomas Penn, *The Brothers York: An English Tragedy*

David Abulafia, *The Boundless Sea: A Human History of the Oceans*

Anthony Aguirre, *Cosmological Koans: A Journey to the Heart of Physics*

Orlando Figes, *The Europeans: Three Lives and the Making of a Cosmopolitan Culture*

Naomi Klein, *On Fire: The Burning Case for a Green New Deal*

Anne Boyer, *The Undying: A Meditation on Modern Illness*

Benjamin Moser, *Sontag: Her Life*

Daniel Markovits, *The Meritocracy Trap*

Malcolm Gladwell, *Talking to Strangers: What We Should Know about the People We Don't Know*

Peter Hennessy, *Winds of Change: Britain in the Early Sixties*

John Sellars, *Lessons in Stoicism: What Ancient Philosophers Teach Us about How to Live*

Brendan Simms, *Hitler: Only the World Was Enough*

Hassan Damluji, *The Responsible Globalist: What Citizens of the World Can Learn from Nationalism*

Peter Gatrell, *The Unsettling of Europe: The Great Migration, 1945 to the Present*

Justin Marozzi, *Islamic Empires: Fifteen Cities that Define a Civilization*

Bruce Hood, *Possessed: Why We Want More Than We Need*

Susan Neiman, *Learning from the Germans: Confronting Race and the Memory of Evil*

Donald D. Hoffman, *The Case Against Reality: How Evolution Hid the Truth from Our Eyes*

Frank Close, *Trinity: The Treachery and Pursuit of the Most Dangerous Spy in History*

Richard M. Eaton, *India in the Persianate Age: 1000-1765*

Janet L. Nelson, *King and Emperor: A New Life of Charlemagne*

Philip Mansel, *King of the World: The Life of Louis XIV*

Donald Sassoon, *The Anxious Triumph: A Global History of Capitalism, 1860-1914*

Elliot Ackerman, *Places and Names: On War, Revolution and Returning*

Jonathan Aldred, *Licence to be Bad: How Economics Corrupted Us*

Johny Pitts, *Afropean: Notes from Black Europe*

Walt Odets, *Out of the Shadows: Reimagining Gay Men's Lives*

James Lovelock, *Novacene: The Coming Age of Hyperintelligence*

Mark B. Smith, *The Russia Anxiety: And How History Can Resolve It*

Stella Tillyard, *George IV: King in Waiting*

Jonathan Rée, *Witcraft: The Invention of Philosophy in English*

Jared Diamond, *Upheaval: How Nations Cope with Crisis and Change*

David Wallace-Wells, *The Uninhabitable Earth: A Story of the Future*

Randolph M. Nesse, *Good Reasons for Bad Feelings: Insights from the Frontier of Evolutionary Psychiatry*

Anand Giridharadas, *Winners Take All: The Elite Charade of Changing the World*

Richard Bassett, *Last Days in Old Europe: Triste '79, Vienna '85, Prague '89*

Paul Davies, *The Demon in the Machine: How Hidden Webs of Information Are Finally Solving the Mystery of Life*

Toby Green, *A Fistful of Shells: West Africa from the Rise of the Slave Trade to the Age of Revolution*

Paul Dolan, *Happy Ever After: Escaping the Myth of The Perfect Life*

Sunil Amrith, *Unruly Waters: How Mountain Rivers and Monsoons Have Shaped South Asia's History*

Christopher Harding, *Japan Story: In Search of a Nation, 1850 to the Present*

Timothy Day, *I Saw Eternity the Other Night: King's College, Cambridge, and an English Singing Style*

Richard Abels, *Aethelred the Unready: The Failed King*

Eric Kaufmann, *Whiteshift: Populism, Immigration and the Future of White Majorities*

Alan Greenspan and Adrian Wooldridge, *Capitalism in America: A History*

Philip Hensher, *The Penguin Book of the Contemporary British Short Story*

Paul Collier, *The Future of Capitalism: Facing the New Anxieties*

Andrew Roberts, *Churchill: Walking With Destiny*

Tim Flannery, *Europe: A Natural History*

T. M. Devine, *The Scottish Clearances: A History of the Dispossessed, 1600-1900*

Robert Plomin, *Blueprint: How DNA Makes Us Who We Are*

Michael Lewis, *The Fifth Risk: Undoing Democracy*

Diarmaid MacCulloch, *Thomas Cromwell: A Life*

Ramachandra Guha, *Gandhi: 1914-1948*

Slavoj Žižek, *Like a Thief in Broad Daylight: Power in the Era of Post-Humanity*

Neil MacGregor, *Living with the Gods: On Beliefs and Peoples*

Peter Biskind, *The Sky is Falling: How Vampires, Zombies, Androids and Superheroes Made America Great for Extremism*

Robert Skidelsky, *Money and Government: A Challenge to Mainstream Economics*

Helen Parr, *Our Boys: The Story of a Paratrooper*

David Gilmour, *The British in India: Three Centuries of Ambition and Experience*

Jonathan Haidt and Greg Lukianoff, *The Coddling of the American Mind: How Good Intentions and Bad Ideas are Setting up a Generation for Failure*

Ian Kershaw, *Roller-Coaster: Europe, 1950-2017*

Adam Tooze, *Crashed: How a Decade of Financial Crises Changed the World*

Edmund King, *Henry I: The Father of His People*

Lilia M. Schwarcz and Heloisa M. Starling, *Brazil: A Biography*